COPING WITH
CROHN'S
The Pain & The Laughter

Sonia B. Glover

COPING WITH CROHN'S
The Pain & The Laughter

Sonia B. Glover

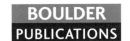

Portugal Cove-St. Philip's, NL
2007

© 2007, Sonia B. Glover

We acknowledge the financial support of the Government of Newfoundland
and Labrador through the Department of Tourism, Culture
and Recreation for our publishing program.

Published by
BOULDER PUBLICATIONS
11 Boulder Lane
Portugal Cove-St. Philip's, NL
A1M 2K1

Cover photo by Sheila O'Leary
Cover design by Vanessa Stockley
Layout by Todd Manning

Printed in Canada

Library and Archives Canada Cataloguing in Publication

Glover, Sonia
    Coping with Crohn's: The Pain and The Laughter / Sonia Glover.

ISBN 978-0-9738501-8-5

    1. Crohn's Disease – Patients – Biography. 2. Crohn's Disease – Popular works.
I. Title.

RC862.E52G56 2007   362.196'3445'0092   C2007-901515-8

This book is dedicated to my friend and cousin, Lorelei Collins,
who died on September 20, 1984, two days before her eighteenth birthday.
Lorelei was a fighter, just as I am.
Her memory lives on.

Together Someday

It happened so fast, I didn't get the chance to say good-bye
We shared so much together, why did you have to die?

You're so special, my cousin and friend
You wanted to be a nurse and I'd be a broadcaster
You never got the chance to fulfill your dream
Well, I'll be graduating in May
If only you could be here when I do
I know you'd be proud of me that day

We were friends since childhood; the memories are endless
The good times and the bad will always be precious
It's been a year and a half now, and I still can't believe you're gone
I promise I'll be looking for you someday

I put this rose upon your chest as a reminder of my love
I pray that God will keep you safe up above
Someday we'll be together again
I really miss you, my friend.

(A tribute to Lorelei, written in 1986)

THANKS

I wish to extend a heartfelt thanks to Christa Skinner, Gerald Poole, Michelle Phillips, Dianne Janes, Beverly Swackhamer, Roxanne White, Adam Hapgood, and my mother, Frances Glover, for being a part of this book and sharing your testimonials. You are heroes.

Thanks to my loving husband Paul for his unwavering support, and to my family for always being there. A special thank you to my friend Kathy Dicks-Peyton for assisting me with the editing of the first draft of the book and for being my sounding board during this project. Thanks to Dr. Jacqueline Elliott, BN, MD, CCFP, for taking the interest and time to review the book. Thank you to my communications colleagues, past and present, for your encouragement. And, a heartfelt thank you to all of my wonderful friends for believing in me. I cherish each one of you.

INTRODUCTION

We all have dreams and goals that direct our lives. One of my dreams was to write a book. During my school days I loved to write, especially poems. I won my first writing contest in 1979, the *What Does Christmas Mean to Me?* competition in *The Beacon* newspaper in Gander. My article was nowhere near a masterpiece, but seeing it, and my name, published in the community newspaper was a proud moment for me at the age of thirteen. I remember an ad in a magazine offering a free book about writing and publishing a manuscript. The book was *The Rogue of Publishers Row* by Ed Uhlan. I eagerly ordered it and received a copy in the mail. I was still a teenager and didn't even understand some of the words in the book, but it piqued my interest in becoming a published writer.

Writing a book, however, was a far cry from writing poems or entering a local writing contest. Living in a small town in rural Newfoundland and Labrador I soon realized that there were more important things I needed to focus on. I had to finish high school and then concentrate on my post-secondary education. I was determined to work in journalism or public relations. I knew that one day, though, the time would be right for me to write a book.

In the fall of 1987 I was diagnosed with a form of Inflammatory Bowel Disease (IBD) called Crohn's disease – the other form is ulcerative colitis. I was 21. With my diagnosis came very painful and trying times. I was a young woman just starting a career, and being told that I had Crohn's disease, which I knew very little about, was devastating. It would change me forever. It was through my adjustment to a new life with Crohn's disease, and the fear of not being able to pursue my career, that I realized I needed to tell my story. After my diagnosis, the pain and trauma continued to grip my life, and in going through such an ordeal I realized that this was the book I had been waiting to write.

The principal reason for pursuing this book goes deeper than fulfilling a career goal. It became personal. I saw it as a mission. I wanted to write a book to educate the public about what a sufferer of

Crohn's disease goes through. I wanted people to understand the pain and frustration of living with this disease. I also wanted to help others who are suffering, often in silence.

In addition to my own story, which focuses primarily on the many years of pain before I was diagnosed and about three years after being diagnosed when I tried to get my life and career back on track, this book also contains testimonials from other brave people who are living with Crohn's disease. They share some intimate moments and thoughts about coping with such a painful illness. My mother tells her story from a family's perspective – the stress and worry that a family goes through watching a loved one battle a frustrating and chronic disease. I was not the only one impacted by this atrocious and painful bowel disease; my family also felt the pain, emotionally. It didn't take long after my diagnosis for me to realize the toll this disease was having on the people who loved me.

The number of Crohn's disease and ulcerative colitis cases continues to grow in Canada. Close to 200,000 Canadians suffer from one of these diseases, which can hit at any age. It is not known how many sufferers of IBD there are in Newfoundland and Labrador, but it is estimated to be in the thousands. The general public does not talk about IBD as it does other diseases. And, given the nature of the illness, many sufferers feel ashamed to talk about their bowel problems. IBD is a debilitating and often humiliating disease that usually requires a significant life adjustment. It has no known cause or cure.

While strides have been made in increasing public awareness of IBD, the stigma associated with bowel disease must be eliminated. It is essential to foster a greater awareness and understanding of the impact of Crohn's disease and ulcerative colitis – this book attempts to do this.

My story is not only about pain and suffering; it is also about a positive attitude, strength, laughter, determination, and the value of family and friends. It is meant to educate the public about IBD, and to encourage people no matter what their illness. If this book inspires even one person, then my writing it will have been worthwhile.

CHAPTER ONE

Childhood Sickness

*W*hen I was about nine years old I started to get sick often – at least more often than a typical child my age – with frequent stomach aches, pains in my side, and vomiting. It was a difficult time in my young life. Besides my health problems, which I first experienced a few years previous to this, I was also going through a family break-up. It was only a few days before Christmas in 1976 when it became official – my parents were separating. It was a difficult time for the entire family. I was obviously hurt, but mostly confused. I knew my parents were having problems, but I didn't think it had gotten to that point. I was young, impressionable, and starting to appreciate the things we did as a family.

My sister Dana, at the age of five, was too young to grasp what was happening. My brother Dirk, a year and a half older than me, kept to himself and was not the emotional type. He always displayed a "strong boy" image. The family situation became stressful for everyone, especially Mom.

It wasn't long after my parents separated that the pain in my stomach became worse and I often vomited after eating my meals. The pain, which usually led to vomiting, was sharp and quick, as if someone was jabbing me every few minutes. When the pain stopped, I immediately braced for the next jab – it was torture. Vomiting actually gave me some relief. I knew, though, that when I ate again, the torture would likely resume. The continuous vomiting also made my stomach muscles burn and ache, and my throat was sore from frequent gagging and coughing. Every time I vomited, I felt as though I was choking to death.

Mom decided to take me to a doctor. It was the beginning of many such visits. She was told by several doctors that it wasn't anything serious. They told her I had stomach flu, a nervous stomach, bowel spasms, or maybe something I ate did not agree with me. One doctor gave me Gravol and said I would be fine. But the vomiting and pain continued. Mom felt helpless. She became increasingly concerned and frustrated. She was convinced that there was something terribly wrong with me and she was determined to prove it.

At one point, I threw up every day for an entire month. Mom marked off each episode on the calendar, which she then brought to the doctor. She insisted that I see a specialist. An appointment was made with a specialist and a number of tests, including X-rays, were ordered. The tests showed that I was suffering from a stomach ulcer. I was prescribed medication to treat the ulcer and put on a strict diet. I was not allowed to eat greasy or fatty foods, such as french fries and hamburgers. The list that outlined what I should not eat seemed endless. My restricted diet was upsetting. I wanted to be a normal child.

My First Night in Hospital

I was admitted to the James Paton Memorial Hospital in Gander around the same time I was diagnosed with an ulcer. All of a sudden one Saturday morning, I felt weak and had severe pain in my stomach and side. I remember bending over in pain for a long time and staring at the green carpet on our living room floor. Uncle Clune drove us to the hospital in Gander. The one-hour drive from Hare Bay to Gander seemed endless. Even worse, Mom seemed angry. Was she mad at me?, I wondered. Maybe I was doing something wrong. I certainly couldn't help it if I was sick. I felt guilty. But Mom didn't know how to deal with all that was going on – family problems, my sickness – she wasn't angry with me, she was angry at the world.

When the doctor said I had to be admitted to the hospital, I was scared. I cried uncontrollably and begged Uncle Clune not to leave me. It was so painful for him to see me cry that he could not even look me in the eye. Despite my pleas, there was nothing that he could do; I had to stay in the hospital. I'll never forget watching Uncle Clune and Mom leave my bedside and walk down the hall to the elevator. I felt so alone. I had flashbacks of the times I got homesick when I stayed at my grandmother's house, which was only next door to ours. If I was afraid to spend a night at my grandmother's house, then I thought I would never be able to stay in the hospital by myself. But, I did; I got through it. After a few days in the hospital the pain in my stomach eased, and the hospital stay became more pleasant. I even made new friends. When Mom came to bring me home, I didn't want to leave the hospital. I felt safe there. I was afraid that as soon as I got home, the pain would return.

A Mother's Helplessness

I continued to be cautious about my eating habits, and while it was assumed that my sickness was related to a stomach ulcer, I felt it might be something more serious. I often missed days at school. It became routine for me to wake up at night with an ache in my stomach, and Mom would give me a hot peppermint drink, which eased the pain for a while. However, Mom was becoming extremely frustrated. She felt helpless as she watched me in such anguish; she wished that she could take away my pain. She often said that she wished she could just snap her fingers and end the torment for both of us. Mom depended on a bottle of peppermint to get me through another night without too much pain. At first she would ask me if I wanted a peppermint drink, but eventually she stopped asking. She automatically gave it to me as soon as she heard me call her name in the middle of the night – the peppermint became her saviour. Mom had a bottle of peppermint in our medicine cabinet for as long as I could remember. I did not understand at the time why the peppermint mixture was so effective in easing my stomach ache – all that Mom would ever say was "Peppermint is good for your stomach."

I discovered a few years later that peppermint has long been known for its medicinal properties. The active ingredients in peppermint, menthol and methyl salicylate, have a calming effect on the stomach and intestinal tract. Peppermint soothes the gastrointestinal tract by relaxing the muscles in the intestinal wall, and is commonly used to relieve upset stomach and to reduce abdominal cramps. Its effect on me seemed magical.

As time went by the pain became sporadic, but, if I felt any pain, I always concluded that it was my ulcer and I would re-commit myself to being extra careful with my diet. I remember eating sandwiches without mayonnaise and that Mom would boil bologna for me instead of frying it. I loved bologna, and, as boring as boiled bologna was, it didn't hurt my stomach, and I ate lots of it, as my diet was limited. When my stomach aches got particularly painful, I ate crackers. Dry crackers also eased the pain.

It became even more apparent to me that there might be something more seriously wrong with me than a stomach ulcer. The oddest things irritated my stomach and nauseated me. When I brushed my teeth, the toothpaste hurt, as did mouthwash. At first I didn't tell Mom that brushing my teeth hurt my stomach because she was already worried enough about my illness, so I told Dad. I recall driving to Gander with Dad when I was about ten or eleven. We were in his car outside the medical clinic, waiting for a relative. I was sitting in the back seat and I asked Dad if mouthwash hurt his stomach. He said no. I told him that when I used mouthwash it made my stomach ache. He didn't seem to think it was anything for me to worry about – he didn't say so, at least. I don't know what prompted me to tell Dad then. Maybe it was being outside the medical clinic that made me think about my health issues. Or maybe I was trying to use the opportunity that day to open up to my father and, in a nonchalant way, tell him that I was concerned about my stomach and wanted someone to talk to about it. I did not want to put any more worry on Mom. I felt like I had become a burden on her.

I didn't press the issue any further with Dad. But when Dad told me his stomach didn't hurt from using toothpaste or mouthwash, I thought that it shouldn't be normal for me. I eventually told Mom. Nothing about my health surprised her at that point. Mom just added the toothpaste and mouthwash to her already long list of reasons why she believed there was something seriously wrong with me. I felt guilty after I told her because I knew that it added to the anxiety and frustration that she was already experiencing as she tried her best to take care of her sick child.

Each time I brushed my teeth I prayed that the stomach discomfort would stay away, but most times I was out of luck. I knew I could not stop brushing my teeth, so I decided to use mouthwash less frequently to alleviate some of the pain.

A Teenager's Stomach Pain

I can't remember getting really sick again until I was about fourteen. One Saturday morning a strange feeling came over me. Mom had gone to the grocery store while Dirk, Dana, and I stayed at home. I was in the bathroom, standing near the sink, when I became weak. Sweat began pouring down my face. I thought I was dying. Things got blurry and I felt weaker. All I thought about was wishing someone would get me to a bed so I could lie down. Then a peaceful feeling came over me. I was ready to fall asleep and never wake up again.

The next thing I remember, Mom was hitting my hand. I was in my bed, but I didn't remember how I got there – my mind was blank. At Mom's insistence I was taken to the hospital that day – this time the doctor said I had stomach flu and needed rest. Again, we took the doctor's advice, but I still thought there was something else wrong with me.

In addition to several such instances, I was, for the most part, a normal teenager. I had a positive attitude and many friends. My health held up fairly well during high school, except for an occasional pain in my stomach and maybe a few more trips to the bathroom during the day than my classmates because of diarrhea. The pain and frequent bathroom visits were blamed on my stomach ulcer. If I got sick, the doctor told us it was likely the ulcer acting up and I was given medication, including Diovol or Tagamet, for the pain. I tried to ignore the discomfort I often experienced. I was not going to let stomach aches and diarrhea interrupt my teenage years.

My high school days were busy ones for me. I did not let my health hold me back. I was the editor of the yearbook, a member of the Student Council executive, a participant in various sports activities, the captain of the volleyball team, a member of the graduation committee, and I participated in public speaking events.

I entered the Miss Teen Central Newfoundland and Labrador Pageant in 1983 when I was in Grade 11; I was named Miss Congeniality, a title that meant more to me than winning the pageant. Dad was in the audience that night watching me. At that moment, I was the happiest girl on earth. I had no pain in my stomach and the diarrhea held off.

My high school grades were fairly good and I was a happy-go-lucky girl who loved to be around people. While we were not a typical family, we still worked hard to be as normal a family as we could be. We had Mom and Dad – they just weren't in the same house, but they loved us. My parent's divorce made me mature faster than other children my age.

Our family ordeal and my sporadic bouts with sickness as I grew up helped mould my personality and character. I was not a religious person, but I believed that God had a plan for all of us and He would not have let me go through such difficult times if He hadn't thought that I could handle them. From time to time, however, I questioned whether there was a God and asked, Why me? I never imagined, however, that I would face more pain and trauma and that my health would get much worse before it got better.

Before I knew it, I graduated from Grade 12. My friend and cousin Lorelei Collins and I talked about what we would wear on graduation night. Lorelei wanted to wear a long dress; I wanted to wear a short one. We went through our usual rant, as most friends do. Lorelei and I had a special friendship. Lorelei, who suffered from asthma, was often sick during high school; her health issues were much more serious than mine. Little did I know that our excited conversations about high school graduation and our career plans after we graduated would be one of the last conversations we would have.

Graduation night was especially wonderful: I wore a short peach-coloured dress and Lorelei wore a long blue one. Dad and Mom were there. It was the first time in several years that I could be with both of my parents – we were together as a family for this special occasion, and I felt proud to have both of them by my side. I promised myself that I would not think about my illness on my graduation night; I wanted it to be worry-free. I was awarded a plaque for my outstanding contribution to my high school, William Mercer Academy. In the back of my mind that evening, though, was the lingering worry of having to rush off to the bathroom with an attack of diarrhea during dinner or of the food hurting my stomach. Neither occurred. It was a perfect night.

Even though my health held up considerably well during my high school years, I did experience occasional pain and discomfort, such as abdominal cramps and some diarrhea. At times the cramping seemed unbearable; it felt as if something was ripping me from inside out. Some days I thought my stomach would explode. I underwent tests, including an Upper GI Series, which is an X-ray of the esophagus, stomach, and duodenum. This test is performed on a fasting patient after that patient has ingested liquid barium. The worse part of this procedure was drinking the thick, chalky barium. Although the barium was flavoured, it tasted terrible, and I always gagged when I drank it. I always feared that I would vomit before the test was performed, or have to use the bathroom during the test.

The other test, a Barium Enema, is an X-ray of the colon: a plastic tube is inserted into the rectum through the anus, and barium is released into the colon through the tube. The barium coats the lining of the colon and makes it easy to view the colon and determine any irregularities. This test was uncomfortable and made me tense up (especially when the technician accidently hit the pole holding the tube and, for a second, it felt as if the tube would be yanked from my rectum). It was a most unpleasant experience, one that became forever etched in my mind.

Nothing out of the ordinary showed up on either of the tests. Most times when I felt sick, I attributed it to a bad day. I believed that if nothing showed up on these two tests, then there must not be anything seriously wrong with me.

CHAPTER TWO

Not a Typical College Life

*A*round the time of my high school graduation I had to decide about a career. I always wanted to be a journalist, preferably a broadcast reporter, or to work in the communications field. I considered myself a "people" person and I wanted to do something that involved interacting with people; I also loved to write, so I felt that journalism would be a wise career choice.

At the time the only place to study journalism in Newfoundland and Labrador was in Stephenville, on the province's west coast. An applied arts diploma program was offered at the Bay St. George Community College. I could do this program, or leave the province and study journalism outside Newfoundland and Labrador, but I wasn't ready to leave the province, so I decided on Stephenville. After graduation, depending on my health, I would decide if I wanted to further my education or enter the workforce.

In September 1984 I headed to a town I knew little about. I was a determined person, and I viewed my sporadic health problems as minor bumps along the road. I tried to think positive thoughts and I had myself believing that my health would eventually improve. While I was anxious about being away from home, nothing was going to get in my way of graduating from Bay St. George Community College. My friends, including Lorelei, headed east to Memorial University in St. John's, while I travelled west. I would be without friends or family nearby. I had mixed emotions.

The first day of college was daunting. I had never been to Stephenville and didn't know anybody there. I was scared, but excited; I was finally on my own and about to begin two years of post-secondary education. I wanted this experience to be one of the best of my life.

I was in Stephenville only a few weeks when Mom phoned with

devastating news. Lorelei had died of an asthma attack. She had been registering for classes at Memorial University, and, on her way back to her room in residence, she collapsed. Lorelei died two days before her eighteenth birthday. She had always wanted to be a nurse, and throughout our high school days we said that when we graduated from college or university we would look for work together outside Newfoundland and Labrador. We often talked of travelling to different places to work. I could not believe she was gone. Why did God do this?, I wondered.

It took me a long time to come to terms with Lorelei's death and I thought about her often during my first few months in Stephenville. I was trying to settle in at college, I had my health issues on my mind, and I grieved over the death of my close friend and relative. My early college days were emotional, but I used laughter to keep focused and I lived each day concentrating only on "today"; I tried not think about "tomorrow" until it arrived. Lucky for me my stomach aches were infrequent during the first few months of college, which helped me adjust to my new life in Stephenville.

Constant Diarrhea and Nausea

But in the spring of 1985 I became ill again. Almost everything I ate hurt my stomach. I had constant weak spells and made frequent and urgent trips to the bathroom because of diarrhea. At times the pain was so bad that my landlady would offer to help me from the bathroom to my bedroom. I didn't know what was wrong with me. I was also embarrassed because of the diarrhea and the horrible smell it sometimes left in the bathroom. It might not have been as bad as I thought, but for me it was humiliating. Every time I used the bathroom, I made sure the door was closed after I left and I prayed that nobody would go in until the smell was completely gone. I was frequently in a mad panic looking for bathroom spray or a scented bathroom cleaner to clean and disinfect the toilet before I left.

I was scared of what might be wrong, but I was also afraid to see a doctor. I wanted to go home. I would often call Mom or Dad and weep on the phone because I was in so much pain. Although Mom and Dad did not want me to leave college, they always told me that my health was more important than school, and that they would support me if I wanted to return to Hare Bay. On the days when the pain seemed intolerable and I felt as if I could not take it anymore, I would always tell Mom and Dad that I would be on the bus the next morning to come home. But when I got off the phone I always managed to fall asleep and when I awoke the next morning I felt better, and would then decide to stay in Stephenville a while longer, always thinking that tomorrow would be a better day. This scenario became routine. And there was the lingering thought that if I went home I would be considered a failure because I was not tough enough to handle my illness and get through college.

Every time I called home my parents became increasingly worried. I wanted to stop making the calls, but just hearing their voices helped ease the pain. But I also knew they had enough to worry about without listening to me cry, and that they felt helpless about being so far away; so I had to be strong and deal with it.

Hemorrhoids

I finally did see a doctor at the Sir Thomas Roddick Hospital, after much convincing from a friend I had met at college. The doctor told me I had hemorrhoids that needed surgery, and that the hemorrhoids were causing the pain and diarrhea. I was surprised and shocked. My mind was jumbled. There must be another reason for my pain. I felt embarrassed – a young college student who had hemorrhoids? It didn't seem fair. I thought only old people got hemorrhoids.

The doctor prescribed Metamucil, a powder that had to be mixed with water or juice, often used to control diarrhea and to relieve constipation. How could one remedy be used for both diarrhea and constipation? What if Metamucil made my diarrhea worse? What if I became constipated and this then caused more stomach pain? Many questions went through my mind, but, in the end, the Metamucil slowed down my bowel movements, which provided me with some relief; I was grateful for that.

I was not prepared to have surgery in Stephenville. In fact, I wasn't prepared to have surgery at all, especially for hemorrhoids. It sounded so gross. But I knew that something had to be done about the pain I was experiencing, and, if this would help, then I had to have surgery. I asked the doctor at the Sir Thomas Roddick Hospital to send my reports to Gander and to consult with my family doctor. He agreed, so I assumed it was being taken care of and that I would soon be admitted to the James Paton Memorial Hospital in Gander. I left the Stephenville hospital, relieved that the doctor had discovered the reason for my pain and diarrhea, but I was also angry at having to deal with the issue. I should have been concentrating on college, not bloody diarrhea and hemorrhoids.

This hemorrhoidal issue occurred at the time of mid-term exams. I endured the pain, thinking I'd have the surgery after exams, during Easter, and then I wouldn't have to miss classes. I feared my sickness would affect my studies and I could not afford to fail. I got through my exams without too much agony and I headed home to Hare Bay for the Easter break. My mind was preoccupied with the hemorrhoidal surgery and I thought of the extreme pain and discomfort I would likely experience after surgery. I also thought about what it would be like to be pain-free if the surgery was a success.

When I met with Dr. Daniel Hewitt in Gander, he said he didn't know anything about the hemorrhoids. My discussion with him that day was the first time he had heard of it. I couldn't believe it. What had happened to my conversation with the doctor in Stephenville who said he would contact a doctor in Gander? Although I was frustrated, I passed it off as a misunderstanding or miscommunication. But I was frustrated because it seemed that every doctor I saw, even when I was a young girl, gave me a different explanation for my illness. I started to question the medical system. Why couldn't things be simple?

Fissure Surgery

I explained to Dr. Hewitt that I was in severe pain and described what had happened to me in Stephenville. I begged him to find out what was wrong with me. How could I get through college if these health issues persisted? He examined me and told me that I did not have hemorrhoids, but, rather, a fissure – a tear in the skin of the anal passage. A fissure is very painful and can sometimes cause diarrhea. It is most painful during and after a bowel movement. I learned later that fissures are common in people with an Inflammatory Bowel Disease (IBD).

The information that Dr. Hewitt gave me explained the pain I had in Stephenville, especially the pain I experienced after a bowel movement. Sometimes I could hardly walk afterwards because the diarrhea was so severe and frequent that my anus became very sore. Frequent bouts of diarrhea left me feeling weak; it drained considerable energy from my body. The doctor explained that the fissure had to be repaired, so I still needed surgery. I was fed up with my health problems and had a gnawing feeling that even after this surgery these problems would not be over. Although repairing the fissure would alleviate the diarrhea, I was still concerned about the unpredictable bouts of nausea and vomiting that I often endured.

The thought of having surgery terrified me. I was admitted to the James Paton Memorial Hospital and spent Easter Sunday in a hospital bed, in severe pain. The doctors said the surgery was a success, but I was in great discomfort, especially during sitz baths. A sitz bath is often required following surgery in the area of the rectum to ease the pain and discomfort, and helps with the healing. A sitz bath is not a full body bath. Only my buttocks and pelvic area were submerged in warm water or a saline solution. The sitz baths were boring and uncomfortable from sitting in one spot, but they usually only lasted about half an hour and they were effective in healing the rectal area.

The most painful and memorable experience from this surgery was the removal of the packing placed in my rectum to help with the healing of the wound. When it was time to remove the packing, the process was not as easy as it was supposed to be. Despite several attempts by several nurses, the packing would not come out. Mom was horrified to witness my pain as nurse after nurse tried to pull out the packing. The unsuccessful attempts meant I had to sit longer in a sitz bath to soften the rectal area as much as possible. My whole body was throbbing and I wanted everyone to leave me alone. I could not tolerate my rectum being touched anymore – it became embarrassing. After a longer-than-normal sitz bath another attempt was made and a nurse was finally able to remove the packing. It was a huge relief, but I also felt as though every bit of pride I had was snatched from me that day.

Although the surgery had been a success, I still felt a little depressed. It was Easter weekend, but I was not in a holiday mood – I wanted to be home enjoying a delicious turkey dinner with my family. My friend from journalism class and boarding-house roommate, Kathy Dicks, sent me a get-well ornament and card. Her thoughtfulness lifted my spirits. Kathy had witnessed my many trips to the bathroom, as well as my loneliness from being so far away from home and dealing with my sickness on my own. Her encouragement enabled me to get through frustrating times and I valued her support, as well as that of all my new college friends.

I was finally discharged from hospital. After a few days of considerable discomfort, I was back on my feet again. I could not believe that I wasn't in any pain, and I thought my days of misery were over. When I left the hospital I returned to college where I had much catching up to do. I wasn't up to travelling on a bus back to Stephenville by myself, which would take a gruelling eight hours, so Mom and her friend Harrison drove me back. The trip by car was faster and much more comfortable than a bus trip.

Back in Stephenville I was happy that the pain had almost disappeared, and the trips to the bathroom were less frequent, but I still felt I was using the bathroom more often than a healthy person would, and I still experienced occasional nausea. I tried not to think about it. I felt one hundred percent better than I had before the surgery.

Summer Break

My summer break began with on-the-job training. The journalism program required all of its students to do a two-week on-the-job training program at a company of their choice, if the company agreed to participate. Since I had an interest in radio broadcasting, 1010 CFYQ radio station in Gander was where I wanted to do my training. The station, owned by CHUM Ltd., agreed. I was excited and two weeks of training convinced me that working in radio was what I wanted to do. The staff at the station treated me well. I longed for the day when I would have a full-time job in broadcasting, and, who knows, maybe even in television.

I was sick only one day during my training. During that episode I felt weak and had to leave work one morning because of constant diarrhea. My on-the-job training finished in early June 1985. I had learned a great deal in just two weeks; I was proud of myself and felt confident that I fit into the broadcasting environment. I was also pleased that my health held up and that the staff were understanding about the one day I was sick.

But before I returned to Stephenville in September for my last year of college, I babysat for my cousin in the Goulds, just outside St. John's, for two months to earn some extra money. During that time it was unusual if I did not have diarrhea after I ate. And there were too many stomach aches. I often lay awake at night, crying in my bed, wishing the pain would stop. I thought about hot peppermint, which used to ease my pain. Even though I told my cousin I wasn't feeling well, I did not complain much and certainly did not believe I needed to see a doctor. I thought my pain was probably caused by the food I was eating.

Except for a few episodes of stomach ache and diarrhea, the summer of 1985 was good. I had fun and made new friends, and I concentrated more on enjoying new friendships than counting the number of times I used the bathroom. But I could not stay away from doctors. I had to be admitted to St. Clare's Mercy Hospital, this time to have a painful cyst removed. It wasn't serious, but having to see more doctors made me want to scream. I was only nineteen and I had already had my share of visits to hospitals and doctors. I often felt discouraged about my health, and thoughts of not returning to Stephenville briefly crossed my mind. But I knew that if I didn't return to college, I would regret it. I was not a quitter.

DIANNE JANES
ST. JOHN'S
AGE: 48

At the age of 21 with a newborn baby I became very ill – loss of appetite, loss of weight, and severe abdominal pain. It took sixteen months to be diagnosed with Crohn's disease. This was quickly followed by hospitalization and a major bowel resection. I returned home to my husband and son after a seven-week hospital stay weighing just 68 pounds. I bounced back and remained well for eight wonderful years and quickly learned that there was life with Crohn's disease. In the years that followed I have endured five more surgeries and many flare-ups and hospital stays for drug treatment for Crohn's.

The flip side of this is that coping comes down to a very personal level. Personally I take many chances; what do I have to lose, a little pride, perhaps, but that's OK. Life is short and I plan to live it to the fullest. Despite all of my suffering with Crohn's disease, God has blessed my life ten-fold. I have met an amazing array of friends through the Crohn's and Colitis Foundation of Canada (CCFC). I have been a volunteer for 27 years now and have raised funds for this organization whose mission is To Find the Cure!

The hardest thing for me as a Crohn's sufferer is that Crohn's is a masked, hidden disease that is hardly talked about openly and publicly. With increased awareness, this is improving every day. The fact that you are taking horrible drugs, such as Prednisone, and have tons of sometimes unwanted weight on your body, people automatically assume you are perfectly fine. Sometimes I try to explain how this works, but for the most part they don't understand and often doubt you. But I always persevere.

Despite having this horrible disease my positive attitude enables me to go, go, go on good days and make the very best of bad ones. Having a strong support base also goes a long way, and I have the best.

CHAPTER THREE

Returning to College

*I*n September 1985 I stood in line to register for my final year of the journalism program. The second year was more difficult than the first year and I had a heavier workload. In addition to attending classes and studying at night, I spent considerable time working on the college newspaper and with the college radio station.

The first half of my second year was good, health-wise, but that changed near the end of the second term. I was busy as editor of the college yearbook and getting ready for graduation. Many nights as we worked on the yearbook I had to leave early and go to my room in the residence because I felt so weak. Most times I did not tell my friends how sick I really was; I kept it to myself. I always put on a brave face and managed to display my upbeat personality. I still did not know what was wrong with me. I only knew that I was miserable and the bathroom was becoming my second home. Thoughts of Lorelei had often helped lift my spirits on the days I sat in class worrying about my health and what I might face in the future.

In February 1986, I entered the Miss Snow Queen pageant as part of the annual Stephenville Winter Carnival. I read a short poem about Lorelei during the talent segment of the pageant. I was not crowned Miss Snow Queen, but I was named Miss Congeniality. I did feel like the lucky one that night, though, because I felt that I had Lorelei back in my life. For a few moments I entered into a world with only warm thoughts of Lorelei. There was no pain or frustration; it was just Lorelei and I, like it used to be. That night, like many times before, I drew strength from her memory to help keep me determined to graduate from college, despite my health problems.

I was using the bathroom so much that I started to feel embarrassed. Some mornings I got up at sunrise to ensure I got to the bathroom before anyone else. I wanted to avoid the humiliation of using the toilet when other students were in the bathroom. I was always looking for infrequently used bathrooms around campus – those not located in a high traffic area. I always kept matches in my pocket which I would light to mask the smell, and I often carried a small bottle of cheap spray perfume. I prayed each time that I went to a bathroom that if the lighted matches didn't work, the perfume would. A deserted bathroom was a haven. Although nobody was around and I could use the bathroom in peace and without humiliation, I felt all alone. What kind of life was this?, I asked myself.

Increasing Frustration

One day as I searched for an empty campus bathroom, I hit a low point. I had become so agitated trying to find a vacant bathroom that when I finally found one I went into a stall, sat on the toilet, and decided to drink the miniature bottle of vodka I had in my handbag (I planned to go out socializing with friends that evening). I used the bathroom and then gulped down the vodka. At first, I felt happy and it was as if the vodka relieved my mind of the intense frustration and worry that had been dragging me down. But then, I felt ashamed and disgusted with myself. It was not my personality to do something so irresponsible and stupid. I thought about Mom and Dad – what would they think of me? The last thing I wanted was to let my parents down. I also knew that alcohol would not take away the pain and I did not want to turn to alcohol as a way to forget my frustrations. Although I only drank a small amount of vodka, I knew that if I continued to engage in such alcoholic escapades I would risk developing an alcohol dependency. I was not about to let that happen. I already felt that my health problems were starting to rule my life – I was not about to let alcohol rule me as well. After that day, I never turned to alcohol when I was feeling stressed about my health.

I missed several classes at the end of the year due to my unpredictable health, and sometimes I found it difficult to catch up. I felt angry and began to question everything: Why should I stay here? Why do I have to put up with this? Should I have even come to Stephenville to attend college? I worked hard to convince myself that I was just going through the stage that some college students go through when they leave home for the first time. I tried to look on the bright side. I was about to graduate. I would soon have a journalism diploma to help me find a job doing something that I had always wanted to do.

Despite my questions and weak moments, I was not going to give up. Thinking positive thoughts gave me the strength to get through another day. I thought about my family and friends, and my mind frequently turned to Lorelei and to how she had been taken from us at such a young age. Thinking of her always put things in perspective – I was thankful to be alive. But I was also frustrated because I didn't understand the source of my health problems. I never let on to anyone how frustrated I really was because I didn't want to put my troubles on anyone else. It took every bit of willpower I had to deal with it and not to let others know how upset I really was. Although I had many friends around me, talked frequently to my family on the phone, and kept a smile on my face, I still felt isolated from the real world. I felt empty on the inside, as if I was trapped in another world with no escape in sight.

CHAPTER FOUR

Struggling to Move Forward

I n May 1986, I walked across the stage at the Arts and Culture
Centre in Stephenville, feeling great pride and accomplishment
in accepting my Diploma in Applied Arts in Journalism. Many times
I thought I'd never get through my final year. I thanked God for giving me the strength to keep going. I had been so sick, especially in my
final year. At this point I didn't care what hurdles I might face in the
future. I thought it couldn't get any worse. I was determined to
become a journalist and to strive to live a happy and healthy life.

After graduation, I worked in Clarenville for the summer as a
reporter and photographer for *The Packet*. I learned much that summer; I was out in the real world working as a reporter, and my time at
the newspaper reaffirmed that I wanted a career in journalism. I loved
dealing with the public, I loved writing, and I enjoyed photography.

But during my time at *The Packet* I used the bathroom frequently and I had a constant stomach ache. The ache was not painful
enough to keep me from working, but it was a torment and discomfort. My greatest wish was to have just one day without a stomach
ache. I knew that going to a doctor would mean tests and I did not
want to face more tests nor hear more theories about my health issues.
Some of my co-workers were aware of my concern about my health
and, even though I did not talk about it much, they often offered
words of encouragement.

By the end of the summer, however, I had become so sick that I
could not avoid going to a doctor. As I suspected, more tests, including a Barium Enema and an Upper GI Series, were ordered. I could
only think, here we go again. Once again, nothing abnormal showed
up. It was not what I wanted to hear. Many questions surrounded my
health issues, but there were no answers.

When I finished at *The Packet* I moved home to Hare Bay with

Mom. I sent resumes to radio and TV stations, and hoped that I would soon get a full-time job. Sitting at home was discouraging; I wanted to be living on my own and proving that I could carry on a normal life and have a stable career. I worried constantly that something serious was wrong with me. What if I got really sick shortly after starting a new job? What if I lost my job because of my sickness? I was driving myself insane thinking about it, even as I fought hard to keep pessimism at bay. Not only did I have a continuous pain in my stomach, I also had a "gut" feeling that there had to be some medical explanation for what I was going through.

Starting My Career

I waited for a phone call for a job interview. I wanted to begin a career and make my parents proud of me. Finally the radio station in Gander where I had done my on-the-job training the previous year offered me a job in their news department. My duties there would include writing news and covering news events. I would be a news anchor. I was so excited; my dream was finally coming true. I started work on October 26, 1986. I was so happy that my health was the last thing on my mind.

My days started between 4:45 and 5:00 a.m. I had to be at work by 6:00 a.m. and my day ended around 2:00 p.m. I was a morning person, so getting up early was not a chore. I loved my job, despite the unconventional hours.

It was fast-paced but rewarding work. It seemed like I was working day and night, but I was lucky to have this job. However, the frequency of my trips to the bathroom started to increase. I especially hated being at functions, such as a banquet or a conference, and having to leave a room filled with people to use the bathroom.

Around Christmas time I felt ill again. Almost every day I was nauseated and I experienced pressure and tightness in my stomach. I was extremely tired all the time and slept whenever I could – I worked and slept. At first I thought I was tired because I got up so early in the mornings and my days were often long. But I could not explain the pain in my stomach, which got worse after I ate. My cousin, with whom I lived, suggested that I see a doctor.

When I could not stand the pain any longer, I made an appointment to see Dr. Hewitt. He prescribed Tagamet to ease the stomach pain, but this medication did not work. Days and weeks went by and I could not eat a full meal without stomach pain or diarrhea. It made me weak, and, like many times before, I often vomited after eating.

A Physical and Mental Drain

A daily routine developed: I ate a regular meal and about five or ten minutes later I'd either throw up or have diarrhea. Several times I woke up in the middle of the night with diarrhea and I would have to rush to the bathroom. Sometimes the diarrhea was so bad that I would wake three or four times at night to use the bathroom. I often found blood in my stool. Some nights I also vomited. These frequent interruptions to my sleep took a physical toll on me. I missed days at work – something I had feared only months before. I didn't want my poor health to ruin my chances of becoming a successful journalist, or any other career path that I might decide to take in the future. At this point, work was more important than my health.

The abdominal pain became more frequent and I often felt as if I could not face another day. My entire body was tired and I was drained physically and mentally. I was also scared. I took the prescribed Tagamet, even though it was not effective. The pain came back, hard; I was saturated with misery. The pain was so bad that I returned to Dr. Hewitt, even though at this point I felt that seeing a doctor would accomplish nothing because no one knew what was wrong with me. It would be the same old story: more tests. That's exactly what happened, and once again the tests showed no abnormality.

CHAPTER FIVE

Suffering Alone

*I*n 1987 my health yo-yoed. I had good days and bad days. It was like tossing a coin to determine what kind of health day I would have. The problem persisted – weakness, stomach aches, and diarrhea. I tried to ignore it. I tried not to complain. I tried not to miss work. I tried to take care of myself, but even that was becoming a chore.

To add to my problems, a cyst which had been removed in 1985 returned. This meant more surgery. Although this problem was unrelated to my stomach and bowel issues, it was still frustrating. Mom was more worried than I was; she could not bear to see me experience more discomfort. I was hospitalized in early April for four days and soon after surgery I returned to work. Proving myself at work and not missing days due to sickness were my priorities. The stomach pain persisted. I worked, and I looked fine on the outside, but inside I was a mess from the physical and emotional torment. In early summer I saw Dr. Hewitt once again. Because Tagamet was not effective, he prescribed another drug, Sulcrate. This drug relieved my stomach pain for a while, but, like Tagamet, the pain kept coming back. It seemed as if medications could only afford me temporary relief.

The pain lingered, and my anger built. Even though I always wore a smile, I was becoming increasingly frustrated about my seemingly hopeless situation. I decided to forget doctors, pain, and pills. I decided to deal with the problem myself. I stayed active throughout the summer and I didn't eat as much as I normally would. It was a simple solution – little or no food meant little or no pain and discomfort, and less frequent diarrhea.

I played the tough girl on the outside, but felt vulnerable on the inside. I needed to explain what I was feeling to someone other than my doctor. I hated to dump my problems on my friends, and I did not want to worry my brother or sister, or upset my parents by telling them how sick I really was. For the most part, I bore the pain alone – at least as much as I could.

I confided in Aunt Glenda, Mom's youngest sister, who also lived in Gander. She insisted that I keep going to my doctor; eventually some doctor would find the source of my pain and misery. But I was sick of doctors. I was sick of X-rays. I was sick of medications. I was sick of being sick. I was too young to be sick. No matter how much Aunt Glenda lectured me, I would not listen.

Job Anxiety

I continued to work hard. I prayed every morning when my alarm went off that I would feel healthy enough to get through another day without too much pain. The pressure in my stomach was becoming so unbearable that I had to wear loose clothing. If anything touched my stomach, it felt like someone was pushing in on my stomach as hard as possible and would not stop. Every day after I finished reading the newscasts I went to my office and cried. I actually read newscasts with my pants undone. The morning DJ kept telling me to go home if I felt sick. I sensed that he didn't believe that I was as sick as I said I was. Didn't anyone believe me? I had already missed several days at work and felt guilty about that, but what could I do? I had an uneasy feeling about the whole situation. I felt isolated at work and I felt as if something terrible was about to happen to me.

Around the end of the summer, the station manager, who was also my supervisor, wanted to meet with me to discuss my illness. I was nervous, as I knew what was coming. He reminded me of the days that I had missed and how this put the station in a difficult situation. He acknowledged that I had been visiting my doctor regularly, yet there was no diagnosis to indicate that I suffered from a serious illness. If my own doctor could not find out what was wrong with me, the company would have another physician examine me. I could not believe that the company would bring in another doctor to determine what was wrong with me. Didn't my supervisor believe me? I felt like I was being accused of a horrible crime, and that my character was being questioned. It was one of the worse moments of my life, and I felt like dying. It seemed that nobody believed I was truly sick.

While he did express some concern for my health, the station manager explained how the news department needed somebody reliable and that I was not dependable as I had been off sick many days. My heart stung and my stomach dropped as I listened to his words. I loved my work. I was a dedicated worker. I would never do anything to ruin my career, a career that had just begun. It hurt me deeply to have to endure this judgement. I needed encouragement, not discouragement.

I felt that I deserved compassion, but I also tried to understand the position of the radio station. I knew that I was the only person working in the newsroom and it was difficult for the station to operate smoothly when I was off sick. I knew they were not trying to intentionally hurt me. I could understand their frustration. However, I did not want to be sick; I was honestly suffering and needed someone to understand what I was going through. I was hoping that the whole ordeal was just a dream and that I would wake up at any moment. It felt as if my entire life was tumbling down around my ears. Nobody understood how seriously ill I was, except for Dr. Hewitt, and he was unable to diagnose my condition.

I assured the station manager that I would be fine. I told him that the reason for my sickness would be found eventually and I would fight to overcome it. I knew I had to work around my illness somehow. I promised not to miss any more days at work – a promise I knew I probably would not be able to keep. But at that point I was determined to crawl to the station on my knees. I never thought, though, that just a few weeks after that meeting I would be rushed to the hospital.

Relentless Pain

I tried hard to keep up my strength and do the best job I could. But I got worse. I threw up frequently and the pain was unbearable. One night in September I had to cover a banquet at Hotel Gander. I actually enjoyed the pork dinner – while I was eating it. When I went to bed that evening, however, I was nauseated and had a terrible pain in my stomach. I managed to fall asleep, but I woke up in the middle of the night with sharp pains. I went to the bathroom to vomit, but could not. The urge to throw up made me weak. I did not know what to do. I prayed that the pain would go away. I literally crawled back to bed, exhausted, and dozed off. My alarm went off a short time later, but I was in no condition to go to work. I called the morning DJ to let him know that I was sick and asked him to let the station manager know that I would be in later in the morning after I had visited the doctor. I was racked with guilt after I made the call and was worried about what would be said to me when I arrived at the station. But I knew I had no choice, despite my promise not to miss any more days at work. I was too sick to even crawl at this point.

I lived next door to a medical clinic, so instead of trying to get an appointment with my family doctor, which would require more time, and I wanted to get to work as soon as possible, I went there. And, I also thought that the clinic doctor might tell me something about my condition that I had not already heard. I described my stomach pain and briefly explained my ongoing problem. The doctor told me that the pain in my stomach could be caused by a number of things, but the only way he could help me was if I had a series of tests done. That's not what I wanted to hear. The same old story once again. All I could think about was that I had spent the past year getting things poked in me, up me, and at me. I knew the doctors were only trying to help, but it seemed as though nothing was being accomplished. I was sick and tired of it all.

However, I tried to stay focused while I was in the doctor's office. I had to believe that eventually an answer to why I was always sick would be found. I told the doctor about the pork I had eaten the previous night, as he asked whether I had eaten anything out of the ordinary. He said possibly the pork wasn't cooked well enough. He also mentioned that some types of food do not agree with certain people. But why was it that most foods I ate didn't agree with me? There had to be a reason. I left the doctor's office very frustrated, and with a note for my boss. I felt more tired with each passing day, and the pressure and pain in my stomach were slowly driving me insane.

CHAPTER SIX

Living a Nightmare

The days and nights that I felt miserable increased in number. It started to become unusual if I did not experience stomach pain at some point during the day. I often dreaded going to bed at night because I knew that an aching stomach would likely wake me, resulting in another sleepless night and exhausting day at work. I was living a never-ending nightmare and I sensed that it would only be a matter of time before I would end up in the hospital's emergency room.

I kept the seriousness of my illness from my family because I didn't want them to worry. Mom and Dad knew I was having problems with my stomach, but they did not know the extent of my illness. Only Aunt Glenda and my roommate knew how sick I really was. My co-workers witnessed my constant trips to the bathroom, my missed days, and my continuous visits to the doctor, but, to be honest, I was never sure what they thought. The meeting with the station manager was never far from my mind, which enhanced my guilty feeling and fear of being considered an annoyance at work because of my health issues.

My constant pain and misery affected my attitude: instead of my usual positive demeanour, I often veered into the cold world of negativity. Some days I hated the world. My personality changed; I found myself judging others more often and I always seemed to be on the defensive. I worried about my health and my job, which I was afraid of losing because I felt nobody believed that I was legitimately sick. Would my dream job be taken away from me? I asked myself this question every day. I felt I was being punished and I was driving myself to a demented state with questions and mixed emotions. I was only 21, but I already felt I had experienced enough turmoil for a lifetime.

My parents were always concerned about my health and reminded me to visit my doctor regularly. I kept them up to date, for the most part, but as I was not living with them, they really did not know the extent of my pain.

The end of September was typical of my life at the time: I was always tired at work and I looked physically drained. After one particularly physically draining day I went straight to bed after work. I felt sick and weak, yet I remember lying on my bed and having a peaceful and relaxed feeling come over me. It was as if I was about to go into an eternal sleep and, for a second, I had no worries or cares. I just wanted to sleep, which I did. It was close to 2:30 p.m. and I did not wake until 5:00 a.m. I had slept for fifteen hours. My roommate had friends over that night, but I had not heard a sound, not even the music.

Still feeling miserable when I got up at 5:00 a.m., I jumped into the shower, hoping that it would make me feel better, but the heat in the bathroom only intensified my weakness and I almost fainted. When I brushed my teeth I felt the familiar pain in my stomach. Toothpaste hurt my stomach. It was so bad that I bent over and held my stomach in my arms. The pain brought tears to my eyes. Why me?, I asked myself again. I wished somebody could help me, but I felt so alone. I needed to talk to somebody, but I did not want to wake my roommate at such an early hour. I prayed that the pain would leave, even for just ten minutes, so that I could get dressed. How I managed to get dressed that morning, I don't know, but I mustered the strength and got to work.

Lingering Guilt

When I arrived, the DJ asked me how I was feeling. I told him I had another rough morning and that I was in a lot of pain again. "Why did you come to work if you are sick?," he asked me. The question upset me. It felt as if I was being a nuisance to everyone. I did not respond, and instead went straight to my office. I prepared newscasts for the morning and re-wrote stories. I performed my regular duties, but it was not a typical morning. I had to unbutton my dress pants to ease the pressure and bloated feeling in my stomach. Reading the newscast with my pants unbuttoned became an everyday occurrence for me at this point.

I managed to get through the morning, but I did not think I could make it through the afternoon. I was weak and nauseated and I prayed for 2:00 p.m. to arrive so that I could go home. Sharp pains in my stomach hit every hour. My office door was ajar and my boss saw me crying. He asked what was wrong. I quickly wiped the tears away and mumbled that I had a stomach ache. His response: "If you're sick, go home." I was embarrassed for crying. I was miserable about my sickness. I felt guilty and, most of all, angry because I did not know what was wrong with me.

I thought my stomach was going to burst open. I wanted to throw up, but couldn't. The pain was always the same. It was as if there was something ripping inside my stomach, trying to get out. But I had to read the news in about fifteen minutes. I pulled myself together; I had to get through the day. It wouldn't be long before I would be home and could rest. This was becoming a typical day for me: a pain-filled morning at work, then sleeping the remainder of the day.

Hospital Bound

I went home after work and crawled into bed. I did not wake until I heard the phone ring. It was Aunt Glenda. I told her I was sick, and, as she had so many times before, she said I should go to the hospital to see a doctor. I would not hear of it. I was sick of seeing doctors. Aunt Glenda then suggested that I should get some fresh air or maybe go to the mall, anything to take my mind off my misery. All I had been doing was working and sleeping. I had been feeling depressed, so maybe some socializing would lift my spirits. We decided to go out somewhere for a quiet drink. Aunt Glenda would pick me up and spend a few hours with me.

Trying to decide what to wear out was maddening because the pressure on my stomach made everything I put on feel several sizes too small. Even light-weight clothing hurt me – it was extremely frustrating. I was in the mood to dress up and go out somewhere in an attempt to try and forget my troubles if only for a few hours, but getting dressed was a problem for me. I also felt unattractive.

We went to a local bar around 8:00 p.m. There wasn't a large crowd there at that hour of the night. I had to get up early for work the next morning, so we planned to stay only a short while. It felt good to be out again. The pain I had been experiencing that day subsided a little, and for a few minutes I was not thinking about work or my sickness. Aunt Glenda and I sat at a table not too far from the washroom. Scouting out washrooms became my first priority whenever I went into a public place.

I had two sips of my drink and a few cheezies when the pain started again. The pressure was getting worse, with sharp pains shooting through my abdomen. It was almost as if I was cursed; I could not enjoy myself for even one hour without getting sick. Aunt Glenda suggested that we go immediately to the hospital, but I said no, hoping the pain would go away. I just wished that I could enjoy a night out and beat this pain for a few hours. Was that too much to ask? I felt nauseated and thought I was going to faint so I told Aunt Glenda I was going to the washroom and if I was not back in ten minutes to come and get me.

As soon as I got inside the bathroom, I vomited continuously. I felt like I was throwing up everything inside of me. I was now in excruciating pain, and I continued to throw up. I must have frightened every woman in the washroom. Sweat was running down my face and my neck and arms felt clammy. I started to cry. Before I knew it, Aunt Glenda was knocking on the door. She did not ask me if I wanted to go to the hospital; she told me I was going – immediately. I was too weak to argue and in no condition to be anywhere except in a hospital bed. I wished this roller-coaster ride I was on would end.

It was about 8:30 p.m. when we arrived at the hospital. The doctor on call examined me and asked me to describe the pain. I did my best – the sharp pains, my weakness, and the constant trips to the bathroom either to throw up or because of diarrhea. I had described my health problems so many times before that I was sick of hearing my own voice and the usual spiel. Looking at the doctor's face, I think he was just as puzzled as I was.

During the questions, Aunt Glenda rubbed my stomach to ease the pain, but it got worse. The doctor gave me medication for pain and decided to run some blood tests. Aunt Glenda explained to him how my sickness had been ongoing for some time and that my family doctor, Dr. Hewitt, was aware of my attacks, but that this one seemed the most severe to date.

When the blood tests were completed, the doctor told me I could go home; there was nothing he could do for me at this time. He advised me to come back in the morning and they would run more tests. I could not believe what I was hearing. I was lying on an examining table, crazy in pain, and he was going to send me home? Aunt Glenda was upset, as was I, but I was too weak to argue. She demanded that my family doctor be made aware of this latest attack and that he be called in to examine me. The doctor said he could not do that because of the hospital policy regarding doctors on call. Aunt Glenda decided she would call Dr. Hewitt herself. There was no way she was going to see me leave that hospital, given my condition.

By this time a couple of hours had passed, and it was almost 10:30 p.m. Aunt Glenda found Dr. Hewitt's number in the phone book and called him. She explained the situation and it wasn't long before he was at the hospital and by my bedside in the emergency unit. Aunt Glenda was still rubbing my stomach as I was being moved to another room in the unit.

Dr. Hewitt asked me what seemed like a million questions. "Please try to explain the kind of pain you are experiencing," he asked. I tried to explain – it was the same old story that I had given him so many times before, but by this time the pain was easing off a little and I just wanted to sleep. During Dr. Hewitt's questioning the nurse brought in the results of my blood tests. My hemoglobin was very low. While a normal hemoglobin is between 120 and 140, mine had dropped to 96. (I did not know this until several days later.)

Then came the obvious. When Dr. Hewitt saw the laboratory results he insisted that I stay in the hospital. I objected to it at first because all I could think was that I had to go to work in a few hours. I was concerned about having to miss yet another day at work. I had already missed too many days. Dr. Hewitt reminded me that there was obviously something seriously wrong with me and tests were needed to determine the problem. Once and for all, we needed to find out what was causing the pain, weakness, vomiting, and diarrhea. Work would have to wait. I was stubborn, but I did realize that my health was more important than work. Besides, I wanted to get rid of this pain – pain that had now taken over my life.

In the end, I had no choice. It was now approaching midnight and I was so exhausted, both physically and mentally, that I didn't really care where I was. Aunt Glenda phone my parents in Hare Bay to let them know what was going on. I was hooked up to an intravenous and I was prescribed pain medication, which was given to me every four hours. Several tests were scheduled for the next morning.

I could not believe I was in the hospital and so sick. I never thought I would ever be in this desperate condition. So many things raced through my mind. It seemed as though my whole life had collapsed and I no longer had any control of it. Lying in the hospital bed that night, all alone, I thought about how lucky people are to have good health. So many people take good health for granted and don't realize how important it is until they go through an eye-opening ordeal themselves.

What was even worse for me that evening was that the nurse who set up my intravenous was the radio station's morning DJ's landlady. "What are you doing in the hospital?," she asked, jokingly. "Aren't you supposed to be on the air in a few hours?" Given how guilty I already felt about losing days at work, I wanted to cry when the nurse told me who she was. Of all the nurses who could have put in my intravenous that night, it had to be the DJ's landlady. I was so emotional about work and my health that all I could think of was her presence that night was another reminder that I could not escape the guilt; it was always with me.

At daybreak, several nurses checked on me; a short time later they wheeled me to my own room on the second floor. I was drowsy from the needle they had given me for pain. It was going to be a busy day: an Upper GI Series, a Barium Enema, and an Ultra Sound. I was becoming used to these tests.

I was anxious to see Dr. Hewitt and hoped he would be by early to tell me how long I would have to stay in the hospital and what other tests or procedures I would have to undergo. I was waiting impatiently when a nurse came to tell me I was wanted on the telephone. I walked down the hall, dragging my intravenous pole. It was the manager from the radio station. "What happened to you, Sonia?," he asked sympathetically. I found the question a little silly at first, especially since I had been so sick over the past few months and consequently had to miss several days at work. I told him I did not know what was wrong with me, and the doctors didn't know either. I explained to him what happened the night before. He sounded concerned and I think he finally realized how sick I was. I started to cry, and hung up the receiver. I did not have the strength to say good-bye.

Answers, Finally

I felt like a wounded puppy. When Dr. Hewitt arrived, my eyes were bloodshot from crying, and I was depressed. He told me right away that my symptoms – bloody diarrhea, abdominal pain, weight loss, fever, and fatigue – pointed to IBD, but the doctors were not sure. The two forms of IBD – Crohn's disease and ulcerative colitis – cause inflammation of the intestines. Crohn's disease can affect any part of the gastrointestinal tract from the mouth to the anus, while colitis affects only the large bowel (colon). It is not known what causes either of these diseases and there is no known cure for Crohn's disease. The only cure for ulcerative colitis is the surgical removal of the entire colon.

The doctors hoped that the next batch of tests would result in a definitive diagnosis. The news scared me. Would I get cancer if I had IBD? Would the doctors have to remove my intestines? Would I be vomiting and having diarrhea for the rest of my life? I did not know much about IBD. I knew that Dad's sister, Aunt Irene, suffered from IBD and that she was often very sick, but I didn't know much about the full impact of her illness. I tried to shake the many questions out of my head. For now, I was happy that the doctors were making progress with a diagnosis.

My first assignment (that's what I called it) in the hospital was to write down the times and types of my bowel movements, information that the doctors would analyze. I did not want to do it. I felt disgusted as I sat on my hospital bed and wrote descriptions: bloody, extremely mushy, soft, watery, stinky, dark, and light. My stool was never hard and formed like that of a healthy person. I always wondered why. Having to describe every bowel movement was not my idea of recuperating. Besides being repulsed as I studied my stool, I also felt weird. What had my life turned into? After a couple of days, it didn't seem so bad; it could be worse – I could be in the bathroom every day, throwing up. And I had to do whatever it took to help doctors get to the bottom of my health issues. So I figured I may as well have fun with it, view it as a way of improving my writing skills. But I soon realized that there are only so many words to describe my disgusting and abnormal bowel movements. In the end, a few descriptions kept circling in my mind – yucky, gross, repugnant, disgusting, revolting – which, unfortunately, were of no value to the doctors.

Following my stool assignment, my diet was changed. I love eating all foods. I always watched my weight and tried to eat healthy foods, but I like munching on snacks and I enjoy a delicious home-cooked meal. My new diet consisted of low-fat foods, less fibre, and nothing acidic. So, what did that leave me? Not very much, it seemed. But the doctors said eating such foods was not good for my condition (although they still did not know my "condition").

That first morning, just like every other day during my stay in the hospital, wasn't long passing. When visiting hours started, Mom was probably the first visitor to arrive. My family, friends, and co-workers came by to see me and were concerned that my health had reached the point where I had to be hospitalized. Get-well cards, flowers, stuffed animals, and phone calls made me realize people cared about me. The first flowers to arrive were from the staff at the Gander radio station. The bright colourful flowers brought a smile to my face and I felt a sense of peace and love that I had not felt in a long time. With so much support around me, I knew I could get through whatever news the doctor would deliver about my health.

When supper was served, I became nauseated. I was quite hungry, and, for some strange reason, I felt that since I was in the hospital I could eat food without experiencing pain. But before I finished eating my meal, I threw up. I was weak and my stomach hurt, and I felt as if the life was being sucked out of my body. I wanted to go to sleep. Mom called the nurse, who gave me Gravol and a needle for pain. The sweat poured down my face so Mom put cold cloths on my forehead. Over the next several days, I went through many tests and endured considerable pain, as the doctors tried to piece together the puzzle and find the cause of my illness. It would not be soon enough.

The Diagnosis

After about a week in the hospital, and what seemed like one hundred tests later, the doctors concluded that I was indeed suffering from a form of IBD. I was diagnosed with Crohn's disease. I'll never forget the day the internal medicine specialist, Dr. Jeffrey Hiscock, gave me the news. My sister Dana and Dad were in my room when Dr. Hiscock explained the disease and told me, in as nice a way as possible, that I would have to live with this illness for the rest of my life. As he gave me some information about the disease, he was also trying to console me. I was a very unhappy girl. I was confused and dazed as I absorbed the reality that my life would be altered forever.

The specialist advised me, as Dr. Hewitt had, that there is no known cause or cure for Crohn's disease. The disease is treated with different medications, including steroids, for most moderate and severe attacks of Crohn's disease or ulcerative colitis. It is more common for Crohn's sufferers to require steroid therapy throughout their illness than a colitis sufferer. I was told I would have to start taking steroids immediately. When the doctors told me about steroid treatment, I immediately thought of Lorelei. She had taken steroids to control her asthma. She had suffered many side effects, such as developing a balloon-shaped face, but she had not let it get her down; this thought inspired me. I could handle it too.

Then, the issue of surgery. Many IBD sufferers have to undergo surgery, usually as a last resort. I was not yet told that surgery would be necessary for me. I prayed to God that the steroids and other medications would be effective as I did not want to have surgery, but there was no guarantee.

After telling me about the immediate action that had to be taken to get my illness under control, Dr. Hiscock then told me the results of my blood tests. My hemoglobin was low, and had been for quite some time. I remember clearly how he was somewhat apologetic when he gave me the information; he suggested that I should have been aware of this before now. My low hemoglobin (96) was one of the reasons I was always tired and weak.

Starting Treatment

When the specialist left the room, Dr. Hewitt walked in. He explained some of the side effects of steroid use. I would be taking Prednisone. I didn't think that the side effects of any medication would be so bad that I could not cope with it, but there was much I would learn. It became clear that I was not to assume anything, but I was trying to think positively. Dr. Hewitt described Prednisone side effects as visible and invisible, adding that the visible effects caused the most frustration: rounding of the face, reddening of the face, the possibility of facial hair growth, and increased bodily fluid resulting in ankle swelling and a pot belly. Steroids users tend to have an increased appetite, which results in weight gain. Mood changes and night sweats are also common. The doctor explained that all of the side effects would reverse gradually, once Prednisone was discontinued.

The invisible side effects of steroid use were more of a concern to the doctors: softening of the bones, thinning of the skin, and an increased risk of infection. Steroids, such as Prednisone, also tend to raise blood sugar levels and can cause high blood pressure. When Dr. Hewitt finished telling me all of this, he stressed that I might not have all of the side effects he described, but I would likely experience some of them. I was confused and scared. Steroids won't make me eat that much, I thought. I will not get fat from taking Prednisone. I could not imagine having mood swings; I was too happy-go-lucky for that.

Being told I had Crohn's disease was a relief, if nothing else. I had reached a high frustration level not knowing what was wrong with me for such a long time. Mom and Dad were relieved as well. The doctors knew now what they were dealing with and could treat me. I didn't think that Mom could handle any more of my painful attacks – throwing up, stomach pain, and diarrhea. She was not only worried about my physical health, but also about my mental state. She knew how anxious I was about being away from work.

The next step was to meet with a dietician and prepare for some dietary changes. When I was finally diagnosed with Crohn's disease, I was bombarded with information from doctors and nurses as the work began to get my health under control. Some days I felt overwhelmed, but I listened carefully to the doctors; I was willing to do whatever it took to get well again.

CHRISTA SKINNER
NORRIS ARM
AGE: 34

In November 1992, after three years of being ill, undergoing numerous medical tests, and seeing eight specialists, I was diagnosed with Crohn's disease. I was 21. I had no idea what Crohn's was.

During the past thirteen years I have had many ups and downs. I have been prescribed many medications, including Mesasal, Pentasa, Salofalk, Imuran, Methotrexate, and, of course, the infamous Prednisone. I was recently given the green light to take a new drug called Remicade. I hope the Remicade treatment will be successful. I have been hospitalized several times. In 1998 I had a right hemicolectomy, which involved the surgical removal of seventeen inches of my small bowel. I was well for about five years after the surgery.

Having Crohn's has also resulted in being diagnosed with chronic anemia, sacroiliitis, arthritis, fistulas, B_{12} deficiency, and osteopenia. One of the difficult things to understand about Crohn's is how it affects so many other parts of your body. I'm not sure if anyone ever really learns to cope totally with Crohn's disease.

I think the hardest part for me is that there are days when I feel so good I'm not sure if I am in my own body, and then the next day I am tired, constantly using the washroom and feeling totally unwell. My biggest fear is being some place where there are no washroom facilities. I avoid such places. It's just one of the many adjustments I have had to make. Despite it all, I do believe that over time, you adjust your lifestyle to Crohn's – you have no other choice.

I thank God that I have a supportive family, co-workers, and physicians who understand me and the disease. Having Crohn's disease has taught me never to take advantage of my health. I have learned to take one day at a time and cherish the good days as they come. You have to keep on going – no matter what – and never let the disease win.

CHAPTER SEVEN

Altering My Lifestyle

*I*t was Thanksgiving weekend 1987 and I was stuck in a hospital. I didn't like the idea of spending this holiday in a hospital, but I had no choice. Since I really wanted to get out of the hospital, my doctor gave me day passes for the weekend, which meant I was allowed to spend several hours a day outside the hospital.

I first wanted to go to a restaurant to get something delicious to eat – maybe splurge a little. I needed a change from bland hospital food. The first thing I did on my Saturday day pass was go to an Italian restaurant. I thought that having an enjoyable lunch at a restaurant with my family would make me feel like my life was returning to normal. I had been feeling well the past day or two and didn't think a little pasta would hurt me. I had conveniently forgotten my new diet and that I should avoid fatty and spicy foods.

I ordered spaghetti and meatballs with garlic bread and a glass of milk. When our order arrived I felt like a child on Christmas morning; the food tasted so good. But after a few mouthfuls I started to get sharp pains in my stomach and I became nauseated. I felt I was going to faint. People in the restaurant stared at me – I was embarrassed. Would I ever be able to eat in a public restaurant again without getting sick?, I wondered.

Dad got me out of the restaurant as fast as he could. Luckily, there were no police cars around that afternoon, as he drove extremely fast through Gander to get me back to the hospital. I could not believe the effect of a little spaghetti and a bite of garlic bread. The ride to the hospital seemed like forever. I cried all the way to my room.

The nurses were surprised to see me back so soon. It wasn't long before they knew what had happened. They told me right away that I should not have eaten anything spicy, and, basically, I should have known better. Dad was not too impressed either. He was worried about me and I knew he had had a fright. I learned the hard way that I would have to be more careful about what I ate and drank. I crawled into the hospital bed, exhausted from all the commotion. The nurse gave me a needle for pain, and it wasn't long before I fell asleep. After that incident, I knew that my diet would have to change, at least in the short term. And I acknowledged that I would likely have to go through similar experiences before understanding everything about the disease – if that was even possible.

A dietician had given me a sheet of paper outlining all the foods that a person with IBD could or could not eat. I couldn't believe what I was reading. All of the food that I loved could cause the disease to flare up. During our discussion about certain foods that I was not permitted to eat, the dietician made an important point, one that is made to all IBD sufferers: for the most part I would have to experiment with foods before I would know what ones aggravated the disease, and that ultimately I would know what foods my body could accept. The dietician stressed that not all people are affected the same way by the same foods. The simple rule: avoid foods that negatively impacted my Crohn's. And always keep my doctor informed about what I was or was not eating.

After my experience at the restaurant, and armed with the information the dietician had given me, I was afraid to eat anything. I feared that the terrible pain would come back. I wanted a break from abdominal cramps and diarrhea, so I became extremely careful about what foods I ate. At one point my diet consisted of water, milk, pineapple juice, boiled chicken, and cheese and crackers. I constantly drank pineapple juice, which I didn't drink frequently before, as it was the drink that caused me the least pain.

After almost two weeks in the hospital, Dr. Hewitt told me that I could go home. I was elated. Going home meant I was on the road to recovery. I was given a discharge care plan sheet containing the dates and times for my appointments, as well as instructions for my care, and a list of medications, including Prednisone and Zantac. I was reminded of my low residual diet. I was happy to leave the hospital, but I was nervous about my new lifestyle. I especially hoped that this would be the only time I'd spend in hospital being treated for Crohn's disease.

CHAPTER EIGHT

The Gift of Family and Friends

Mom and Dad wanted me to come to Hare Bay for a few days, but I just wanted to go back to my apartment. I wanted to relax and forget about pain, hospitals, and doctors. I wanted a normal routine. I promised them I would take care of myself.

What a sense of relief to walk into my apartment. I would have to take care of myself and follow the doctor's orders, and I made a promise to myself to do everything in my power to stay out of the hospital and keep my disease under control.

I couldn't wait to get back to work. One more week and I'd be back on the air, working at the job I loved. I couldn't imagine having to go through all the pain that I experienced before at work. Maybe now I could keep my pants done up when I read newscasts. I also thought that mentally I would be much stronger because my boss and co-workers now knew I had a legitimate illness and I would no longer have to feel guilty.

Not long after I returned to my apartment my friends started to visit me. Knowing I had supportive friends helped me. Their cards, flowers, words of comfort, phone calls, laughter, and constant offers of help inspired and strengthened me, one day at a time. I believed that God gave us the gift of friendship not only to create happy moments, but also to depend on during tough times.

The first thing I wanted to do, now that I was back home in my apartment, was to cook a delicious meal for myself. I loved to cook and missed it while I was in the hospital. I decided to have boiled chicken with pineapple sauce and rice. I kept my new diet requirements in mind – rice would not hurt my stomach and, surely, boiled chicken would not be greasy; it seemed a perfect meal for my first night home. My roommate was at work, so I was alone in the apartment. I felt so relaxed and good about myself, something I had not felt in a long time. I was thinking about baking, so my spirits must have been up (I hate baking).

What a great meal it was. I had not eaten much in the past few months because it was the only way I could keep the pain at bay. However, as I started to wash the dishes I felt weak and the now-familiar pain returned. I tried to ignore it, thinking it was only natural to have a little pain after a big meal. However, as I lay on my bed, the pain got worse. I could not sleep and sweat profusely. I became nauseated and before I knew it I was in the bathroom, throwing up. For a moment, I felt defeated, like there was no hope. Is this what I have to put up with for the rest of my life?, I asked myself. I managed to get into bed after drinking some cold water, and I eventually fell asleep.

The next morning I asked myself a dozen questions. Wasn't the medication working? Why was I in so much pain again? I had thought that since I was taking medication for a specific illness, everything would be fine. I thought my days of severe pain were over. I was obviously expecting too much too fast. Frightening thoughts crossed my mind: What if I have to go back to the hospital? What if the medication won't work for me? Would I have to face surgery? My mind was cluttered with different scenarios, making me anxious.

I remembered my conversation with the internal specialist, Dr. Hiscock, at the James Paton Memorial Hospital, about surgery, how for some IBD sufferers surgery is not an option – in some cases, patients require an ileostomy or a colostomy, where the lower small intestine (ileum) or the large intestine (colon) is cut and brought to the outside of the body through a hole in front of the abdominal wall. The intestine is then fitted to a plastic bag that collects waste from bowel movements. Ileostomies and colostomies may either be temporary or permanent, depending on the patient's situation.

The thought of such procedures increased my anxiety, and it disgusted me. Eventually, however, I calmed down. After all, I might never need surgery. Perhaps I could avoid it by being more careful with my eating habits. I concluded that the pain I experienced after eating the chicken and rice was likely from the vinegar in the sauce. Bad decision, indeed. I loved vinegar, but I added it to my list of foods not to eat, or to try not to eat. The list would get longer as time passed.

I then decided it was time to go to Hare Bay and I called Mom to tell her I would come home for a few days before I returned to work. Just moments before Mom and her friend Viona arrived at my apartment to get me I had a phone call from my brother Dirk in Winnipeg. He had been worried about me. My brother, who is in the Canadian Armed Forces, had left home at a very young age, and we didn't often get to speak on the phone. The phone call was a simple action, but hearing his voice had a powerful and positive influence on my spirits. I realized more each day the irrefutable impact my family had on me as I coped with my health issues. My family drew closer to me as my illness worsened and the uncertainty about my career continued to haunt me.

The first thing Mom said when she walked into my apartment was, Did you have anything to eat? It was a typical mother's question. I had gone from about 127 pounds to 118 pounds in just a few days. Mom said I looked too skinny, and being skinny, to her, meant I looked sick; adding extra weight would make me look healthier.

The Impact of Steroids

On the day we left my apartment to drive to Hare Bay an uneasy feeling came over me – I felt I would never be back. This uneasy feeling soon faded and was replaced with a warm feeling when I arrived at the trailer where I had grown up. When I met my sister Dana at the door, I felt safe. I went straight to my bedroom to unpack my things and to have a nap. I tired easily, so I lay on my bed for a while. All of a sudden, a sharp pain shot through my stomach and I found myself practically on the floor. I hugged my stomach as I once again tolerated the pain. Mom came running into the room and the first thing she said was, "you should not have been released from the hospital." She rushed to the kitchen to get me a cup of tea. Something hot used to relieve the pain, and, sure enough, it worked again.

That night I experienced my first side effect from Prednisone. I had been asleep for about two hours when I woke up in a cold sweat. It was weird. I was sweating uncontrollably, yet I felt extremely cold, with goose bumps all over my body. I remembered the doctor telling me that people taking steroids frequently experience night sweats.

This side effect could indicate a serious illness and needed to be reported to a doctor. I didn't know how true that was until about two or three nights later when I thought my life was ending. I had not been sleeping well the previous two nights and this one was no different. An odd feeling came over me around 2:00 a.m. When I awoke, I was in agony, hurting from head to toe, my head especially, mainly around my eyes. I didn't know what to do. I called Mom, but she didn't hear me at first. I turned on the light and suddenly became nauseated. My vision blurred and my body ached so much that it hurt just to lie in bed. Despite the pain and nausea I managed to walk into the hall and yelled to Mom as loudly as I could.

I knew I had a fever, but I didn't know what was happening to me; I thought I was dying. My body felt wilted; I didn't have the strength to even raise my arm long enough to take the cold cloths from Mom's hand. She placed cold clothes on my head and suggested that I go to the hospital, but I refused. I was so scared that I didn't want to hear of going back to the hospital. Mom was not impressed with my decision, so she said if I was not feeling better within an hour or so she was going to call Dad and get him to take me to the hospital in Gander.

My eyes, head, back, legs – everything hurt. I could not stop crying, which caused my head to throb harder and faster. Mom lay on the bed with me and rubbed my back and legs to relieve some of the pain. My entire body was one big ache. It felt like my body was on fire and someone was exerting extreme pressure on me. Mom did what she could to make it better.

My mother kept insisting that I see a doctor, but I would not hear of it. By 6:00 a.m. my eyes were swollen from crying all night. I was sweating profusely. Mom kept cold cloths on my face, and rubbed my back and stomach. The pain was so bad it was as if the bed hurt me just by my touching it, so Mom carried me to her room – her bed was a little softer and maybe I would be more comfortable.

I hated the suffering, but I would not give in. I knew the pain had to end at some point. But what was wrong with me? All I could figure was that I was having a negative reaction to the steroids. I could not think of any other reason why I felt like I was dying. I had already

48

been through so much, and I was supposed to be on the road to recovery, not enduring more agony.

I fell asleep around 7:30 a.m., but awoke again at 9:00 a.m. I did not feel much better; my body was drained from trying to fight a force that seemed unconquerable. My eyes were swollen and glossy. I couldn't muster enough strength to lift my head from the pillow. Mom felt frustrated and helpless, but I eventually gave in and agreed to go to Gander to see my doctor. I was too weak to dress myself so Mom had to dress me and even help me brush my teeth. How could a 21-year-old find herself in this situation?, I wondered. I felt like an invalid. What did I do to deserve this misery?

When I arrived at Dr. Hewitt's office, he wanted to admit me to the hospital again. I wasn't impressed with that suggestion since I had only been discharged from the hospital a few days before, and I did not want to be re-admitted. I was angry and I felt cheated by the medical system as I thought I was supposed to be on the road to recovery, not being faced with another possible hospital stay. I asked Dr. Hewitt why I was so sick. He explained that people react differently to drugs, especially steroids. He felt it was probably a side effect of Prednisone, but given that I had gone through such an ordeal the night before, I should stay in the hospital so he could monitor me for a few days. After I pleaded, Dr. Hewitt let me return home on one condition – I would have to report to his office every day for one week. I wasn't thrilled with that idea either, but it was better than being back in the hospital.

I obeyed my doctor's orders and we drove back and forth to Gander every day for a week. My health improved, but not to the extent I had hoped. Again, I expected too much too fast. Dr. Hewitt was very understanding and talked to me about my feelings. He told me to try not to get depressed about my condition; my situation would improve. I will always be grateful for Dr. Hewitt's support. I almost thought of him as a friend instead of a doctor. Having a good patient-doctor relationship is important in coping with Crohn's disease. Dr. Hewitt understood my frustrations with the disease and he knew how anxious I was to get well and return to work. We often discussed how important a successful career was to me, and how I desperately wanted to get on with my life and not be burdened with health problems, especially at such a young age. I sensed that Dr. Hewitt was also frustrated; he was doing the best he could to help get this stubborn disease under control.

An IBD Support Group

In an effort to lift my spirits, Dr. Hewitt suggested that I attend a meeting for people who suffer from IBD, through a national organization called the Canadian Foundation for Ileitis and Colitis (CFIC). This group had an active chapter in Gander. Someone had told me about this support group for people with bowel diseases, but I had dismissed it. Dr. Hewitt thought it would help me if I met other people with IBD and talked with them about similar experiences. He suggested that it might be good therapy and help to relieve some of my frustrations. CFIC is a non-profit organization dedicated to finding the cause of and cure for IBD, and an educational and support group for IBD sufferers.

I now decided to check out the Foundation. I had been reluctant to attend such meetings at first because I was still trying to accept my illness and wasn't ready to talk to strangers about my bowel problems, nor did I want to listen to other people talk about theirs. But I realized this was selfish and stubborn. Maybe I could help someone deal with their pain and frustrations. Despite my pride, I felt I had nothing to lose and much to gain, so I attended a meeting.

After speaking with members of the local chapter, I realized that CFIC could have a positive impact on me. Being a part of this organization would help me cope with my disease, as well as educate me about IBD and, in turn, I could educate others, especially my family and friends. I had always heard of support groups for various medical problems, but I never thought I would ever be a member of one.

Attending a meeting of the Gander chapter of CFIC was a crucial step toward accepting my illness. Such meetings provided all sufferers with an opportunity to help each other cope with the disease. Just knowing you are not alone is a starting point. It was not long before I became an active member and dedicated myself to volunteering for the Foundation. I was soon elected vice-president. The experience solidified my acceptance of my illness – I brushed away my fears and defeatist thoughts about living with Crohn's, and accepted the fact that it was up to me to make a choice about my attitude towards the disease. Almost every day I told myself I could deal with this illness, and that I would do my best to help others. I began to realize that having Crohn's disease wasn't so bad after all.

CHAPTER NINE

Crohn's or Not?

The next important step in controlling and treating my illness was to see a bowel specialist. Not all sufferers of Crohn's disease follow the same path, but Dr. Hewitt recommended that I see a specialist in St. John's. I was not pleased about having to see yet another doctor.

I was scheduled to see a gastroenterologist and internal specialist at the Health Sciences Centre in St. John's on October 26, which happened to be the date of my first-year anniversary with CFYQ radio in Gander. It was a day of mixed emotions for me – I should have been working and celebrating this anniversary with my colleagues. Instead, I prayed that this doctor would help me become well enough to return to work.

I had been on Prednisone less than a month and my face was getting larger and rounder. My whole body felt like a big round balloon. I hated my friends to see me this way. I knew that my friends didn't care how I looked and they would love me anyway, but that did not erase my paranoia. Every time I met with friends, I explained that my condition was only temporary and I would only look like this while I was taking Prednisone. I wanted to promise them that I would look normal again soon. While it wasn't as bad as I made it seem, I did feel abnormal. I desperately wanted to look "me" again. I dreaded to look in the mirror. I saw a stranger with a plump face, a stranger I wanted to go away.

My friend, Rodney Etheridge, who worked with the same radio company that I worked for, picked me up at the bus stop in St. John's. All I could think about was what he was going to say about my round, puffy face, but he didn't even notice it. I immediately told him how upset I was about being on steroids; it was as if I had to tell everybody about the steroid I was taking before they had a chance to make a comment, if at all, about the visible effects of the drug. Maybe I was over-reacting, but I could not control the emotional impact that Prednisone was having on me. Negative thoughts about my appearance dominated my mind.

My visit with the gastroenterologist went as I expected. He wanted my medical background and, of course, he asked routine first-visit questions. I felt like a parrot, always repeating my words. My bowel X-rays had been sent to the gastroenterologist and, after examining me, which included a dreaded anal examination, he left the room to look at my X-rays. When he came back, he told me that, from what he could see on the X-rays, there wasn't enough evidence to definitively state that I was suffering from Crohn's disease. I almost fell off the examining table. Had I heard him correctly? There was obviously something wrong with me, so if it was not Crohn's disease, then what was it? While he said it was quite possible that I was suffering from Crohn's, more X-rays were required to confirm this.

I could not believe it. What is it with all the varying medical views?, I wondered. I took his comments in stride and went back to Hare Bay totally confused. I am sure he did not mean to upset me and he just wanted to be one hundred percent certain that I had Crohn's. As I was leaving his office, he suggested that I come back in a couple of weeks for more tests. I was not thrilled with that suggestion. I wanted to scream, but I knew that screaming would accomplish nothing. Just thinking about having yet more tests, I didn't know whether to laugh or cry – it seemed so surreal.

I returned to Dr. Hewitt for a check-up. He had received the gastroenterologist's report and, just as I thought, Dr. Hewitt did not agree with his suggestion that more tests were needed to confirm Crohn's disease. He saw in my face how disappointed I was at even the thought that there might be a slight chance that I did not have Crohn's. Dr. Hewitt assured me again that, as far as he and the internal specialist who reviewed my X-rays in Gander were concerned, I was suffering from IBD, and he felt that further tests were not necessary. The decision to have more tests was up to me. At first, I felt burdened to have to make such a decision. But then I felt that I was simply being put in a position whereby I had to take control of my own care. I had either to take Dr. Hewitt's word and concentrate on getting my Crohn's under control or undergo more tests.

I had faith in Dr. Hewitt and I trusted him. I had been through more than my share of bowel tests and I did not want to go through any more torment and inconvenience, if it was not necessary. I also believed that getting a second medical opinion would be a wise move, given that my future health was at stake. While some patients hesitate to get a second opinion, for such reasons as fearing that their actions might offend a doctor, I had a nagging feeling that a visit to a second bowel specialist would reinforce what I, and Dr. Hewitt, already believed – that the tests I had undergone, indeed, showed enough evidence to diagnose Crohn's. After I mulled over the issue, I expressed my thoughts to Dr. Hewitt. He then suggested I see another gastroenterologist in St. John's, and I anxiously agreed. He made an appointment for November 26 with Dr. Timothy Higgins. Another new doctor. Dealing with so many doctors became confusing and I wondered what this one would say about my condition. One thing I did not want him to say was that I had to undergo more bowel tests.

I was lucky when Dr. Higgins confirmed that more tests were not needed to confirm Crohn's disease. After reviewing the X-rays, he agreed that I was indeed suffering from Crohn's disease, but he also suggested that I have bowel surgery right away. What? Immediate surgery? Another unexpected recommendation. I had gone from one bowel specialist who said I should get more tests done to be sure that I was suffering from Crohn's disease to another who suggested immediate surgery. I felt I was always riding an emotional roller coaster. Dr. Higgins suggested that the best form of treatment was to undergo surgery as soon as possible to remove the abnormal or inflamed section of my bowel. He made it sound so simple, almost painless. But I was terrified; I stood in a daze as I listened to him speak.

I thought, there's no way I can have surgery now. I did not think I was ready to have surgery yet, if it wasn't an emergency. When I was diagnosed with Crohn's I was told about the possibility of needing surgery, but I never imagined that I would have to face it so soon, if at all. And, Christmas was just around the corner. I didn't want to be hospitalized or recuperating from surgery during the holidays. Many of my friends and family members were coming home and I wanted to spend time with them. Dr. Higgins understood and did not think it would be a problem, given that I was not in a critical state. The surgery would be put off until early in the new year.

.

ADAM HAPGOOD
GOOSE BAY
AGE: 21

My struggle with Crohn's disease has been a long one, with my symptoms beginning at the age of nine. The symptoms were unusual for Crohn's. I was plagued with painful and tender red nodules near the surface of my skin, usually my hands and feet. I had painful swelling as well, which restricted activities like walking and skating. Different drugs were unsuccessful in treating this skin condition. When I was twelve years old, doctors discovered pyoderma gangrenosum on my leg; further tests revealed that I had Crohn's disease. The feeling wasn't one of being frightened, it was more of a relief.

Following a few good years with treatment after my diagnosis, things changed. I reflect regularly on two moments in my life – the passing of a good friend when I was fifteen and, three months later, a ten-week hospital stay. I went to the local hospital in Goose Bay, Labrador, with typical bowel disease complaints. I was admitted and awaited a bed in the old Janeway Children's Hospital in St. John's. A series of tests revealed an abscess and a fistula. Surgery was required. My bowel needed to heal before the operation; this meant complete bowel rest, which turned into nothing to eat for seven weeks.

The beginning of my stay in the hospital was tough. I cried, and asked, "Why me?" But, this soon passed. I decided to make the best of the situation. I befriended the nurses, telling them jokes and pulling pranks, and talked to other patients on the ward. I lived on the cancer ward for about five weeks. This was due to the familiarity that the staff there had with Central Line Intravenous. I had my Central Line in place for five months and during this time I could not take a shower. Today, I sometimes stand in a warm, relaxing shower realizing that there was a time when I could not do this, and such a time may come again.

I remember going for a barium swallow test after several weeks without food. I saw the strawberry-flavoured barium as an exotic drink. Anything with flavour that I could savour was heavenly. On recovery days when I started a liquid diet, warm soup broth or Jello tasted exquisite. Looking back on my time in hospital, some days were hard, but I recall mostly happiness. I think of the good memories. Crohn's disease has taught me to live this way. The disease is terrible, but the only moment we ever have is right now and we must find happiness in it.

I had a couple of symptom-free years; then the summer before I started university, testing showed that the disease was active again. I have now completed almost four years at Memorial University of Newfoundland and would not hesitate to say that Crohn's disease is a better educational device than any book I have yet found. I now take four courses a term, allowing for some down days. I've had to drop courses occasionally due to sickness. This slows down the completion of a degree and can be annoying, but then memories of a well-fought battle and a realization that it must continue come to mind – Crohn's disease only wins the fight if you let it.

Good advice for all Crohn's sufferers is to enjoy the things that are a part of everyday life. I would not wish Crohn's disease on anybody, but for those of us who have been cursed with it, we must also view it as a blessing. We are given a unique perspective on this life and have an opportunity to learn from it. What we can take away from this experience we should pass on to others.

CHAPTER TEN

Preparing for Bowel Surgery

As the Christmas season approached, I dreaded the surgery scheduled for January 18, 1988, at the Grace General Hospital. When I was advised of the date, I immediately thought of my sister Dana, as this date is her birthday. I felt guilty because Mom would be in St. John's with me on that day, and I knew that Dana would worry about me instead of celebrating her seventeenth birthday. If I had my way, I would have changed the surgery date, but I knew that it was not possible nor would it be wise. I needed to regain normal life, and to accelerate my recovery.

As Dr. Higgins had already explained, the surgery would involve the re-sectioning of my bowel: removing the diseased part of my bowel and joining the two healthy ends of the intestine. It seemed simple enough. Painful, but simple. He made it clear, though, that surgery was not a cure for Crohn's disease, and the inflammation could return. It could happen months after surgery, it could happen years after, or it might never happen at all.

All I wanted was the pain to go away and to stop taking Prednisone. My experience with Prednisone had been horrible, especially the irritating side effects of cold night sweats and mood swings. Dr. Higgins told me that my intake of Prednisone would gradually be decreased over the month prior to surgery. In addition to other medications, I had been taking up to eight Prednisone pills a day since my diagnosis in October 1987. This was to be decreased to two a day by the time of my surgery.

My doctors had convinced me that surgery was necessary. I promised to be optimistic; I would once again depend on my positive attitude to get me through. I was anxious to get back to work, however, and it was upsetting to know that having surgery meant being away from work even longer. It bothered me to hear someone else read the news on the radio; it felt as if my job had been stolen from me. I had to accept that my career was now on hold, but I was determined to remain optimistic that with God's guidance I would soon get back to a healthier life and to work. For now, I just had to be patient.

In December I met with Dr. Hiscock at the James Paton Memorial Hospital. He had been briefed on my recent visit with Dr. Higgins. Dr. Hiscock also felt that surgery was a good idea, but he went even further and said I should have it before Christmas. According to him, I probably should have had surgery in October when I was first diagnosed with Crohn's disease. I was adamantly opposed to surgery before Christmas. I explained to him, as I had to Dr. Higgins, that I did not want to be sick or recuperating during the holidays. There was no point in trying to change my mind. I prevailed, and later in the month returned to Dr. Hewitt's office to discuss the pending surgery. He prescribed iron pills as my blood lacked sufficient iron. As the surgery day got closer, my nervousness increased. But, like many times before, Dr. Hewitt told me not to worry; he reassured me that everything would be alright.

Fading Self-Esteem

Christmas soon arrived. The feeling of peace and love was in the air, as friends and family trickled into Hare Bay for the holidays. I was happy to see my friends again but something wasn't quite right. My moods changed constantly and my self-esteem had faded. I hated to look in the mirror because my face was a round balloon.

My family and friends also noticed how different I looked because sometimes I caught them staring at me as if they pitied me. Not only was my face puffy, I was also retaining fluids, both a result of the steroids, and I was gaining weight. The thought of getting fat made me angry. I was hungry all of the time; sometimes my midday snack consisted of six slices of toast and a dessert. I couldn't eat enough Vachon snacks, especially vanilla half-moons, which didn't hurt my stomach. Many times this still did not satisfy my hunger; I often wanted to eat more but forced myself to stop.

I tried to do something, anything, that would make me feel better. I tried to lose the weight by exercising, and I even went to a tanning salon in Gander in the hope that I would feel better about myself if I had a tan. If I looked better, I thought, maybe my self-esteem would follow. Indeed, getting a tan did make me feel better about myself, but only for a short time. Getting a tan did not get to the crux of the issues I was dealing with, like feeling unattractive and experiencing bouts of low self-worth. Mom did not agree with me going to a tanning salon; she felt it was unhealthy and that tanning caused premature aging. Mom made her feelings known, which caused some tense moments between us, but she also tried to understand my desperate need to feel better about myself. And after a while she did not say much, as she knew that her comments would fall on deaf ears.

I woke up night after night with cold sweats due to the Prednisone. I started to think that maybe I should have had the surgery earlier and all of this agony would have been eliminated.

With the holidays over, relatives and friends returned to their homes. I counted the days before my surgery, which I was depending on to reduce my pain and discomfort.

CHAPTER ELEVEN

The Unforgettable Bowel Surgery

I was admitted to the Grace General Hospital the middle of January 1988. I had dreaded this moment for months, and it came faster than I had anticipated. Mom travelled to St. John's with me, and she was by my side throughout the entire ordeal, from 8:00 a.m. to 8:00 p.m. every day for almost two weeks. Since she did not like to ride in elevators, Mom walked up several flights of stairs every morning and back down every evening. By the time I was ready to be discharged I thought that Mom looked sicker than I did; exhaustion and worry had taken a toll on her.

The first few days in the hospital were routine. Tests were ordered – again – and I met with Dr. Higgins and Dr. J.P. Gardiner, the surgeon. They both explained the details of the surgery and how a part of the bowel by my lower right side would be removed. They didn't anticipate any problems and assured me that everything would be fine. They did say, though, that there was always a chance that things could change during surgery when they could better determine the condition of the bowel. Although highly unlikely, the doctors noted that there was always the possibility of the need to perform an ileostomy. I cringed even at the thought of it. I looked over at Mom and her face was white from the shock of hearing this word. It was overwhelming for both of us.

The surgeon indicated on my stomach where he would be operating and said he didn't think that a big incision would be necessary. I half-jokingly said that I would hold him to that, as I didn't want to have an ugly scar on my belly. Any young, single woman wouldn't want an ugly scar on her stomach! The doctors told me that when I awoke from surgery I would be hooked up to several tubes and machines, which was the normal procedure for the type of surgery I was about to have.

When Dr. Higgins and Dr. Gardiner left my room, the anxiety set in and I was scared. Even though Mom would not admit to it, I knew by the look in her eyes that she was just as scared as I was. I could not believe I was in a hospital bed waiting to have a bowel re-section. Prepping for surgery included a bath and my "happy" needle. I had to change into the appropriate cap and gown – what a beauty I was, with a smile on my face that stretched a mile, thanks to the needle. Before I knew it I was wheeled into the operating room, but I felt like I was walking on air. Now if only I could feel this way all of the time, I thought.

I next remember waking up in the recovery room and feeling very cold. I could not stop shivering. The nurses put more blankets on me, and the next time I awoke I was in the Special Care Unit. Mom was by my side, wiping my forehead. I looked at all the tubes around me and wondered if in fact I was hooked up to all of them. Yes, I was; five of them. It was like a dream. Mom said I mumbled something like, What's happening, Mom? or What's going on, Mom?, and then I went back to sleep. She also said I mumbled about pain and suggested someone was hurting me. I was obviously feeling the effects of the anaesthetic.

A Scary Recovery

After a day or two I was alert and understood what was happening around me. It was frightening to see all the tubes hooked up to me – an intravenous, a blood transfusion, a nasogastric tube in my nose going down to my stomach to decompress the stomach after surgery, and a spinal epidural to deaden the area where there was pain – I was virtually in a paralyzed state from the waist down. I got a big fright when I could not feel my legs, but at least I was free from pain while the epidural was in me and morphine was being injected into my body. I was also hooked up to a catheter. What a frightening experience all of this was.

When the nurse got me out of bed after surgery, I had an even greater shock. My entire body hurt; I was as stiff as a frozen fish. I will never forget the terrible pain and a "tearing" feeling in my stomach. It was like someone was ripping the staples out, over and over, and dragging out my suffering as long as possible. It took me some time to build up the nerve to look at my incision. When I did, I could not believe my eyes. I expected just a tiny cut, but, much to my surprise, it looked as if there were about fifty staples in my stomach. The actual count was only half that, but it looked like a lot more. I was probably being egotistical, as I knew what I was going through was probably only minor compared to what others have gone through, but the first thing that came to my mind when I saw the incision was how the doctors had told me it would be small – certainly nothing big and ugly like this. Instead of being happy that the surgery appeared to be a success, I was concerned about how my belly looked. The doctors explained to me later that it is difficult to determine exactly the size of an incision until the surgery is in progress.

The surgery was over and I first concentrated on being able to get in and out of bed, and maybe a short walk with the least amount of pain possible. It was a new challenge. I felt as if I weighed a thousand pounds, and the pain was piercing. As time went by, however, it got easier. I became a stronger woman, walking up and down the hospital hallway in my pretty light green lace-trimmed nightgown and robe that Mom bought for me. (I still have that nightgown.) Several nurses called me a princess. I laughed when they said this; it felt good to laugh.

After a couple of days I was moved out of the Special Care Unit and into a semi-private room. Most of the tubes had been removed, except for the nasogastric and intravenous tubes. During my last night in the Special Care Unit, I woke up around 3:00 or 4:00 a.m., feeling soaking wet. I thought I was bleeding. I panicked and buzzed a nurse. She came immediately and discovered that the nasogastric tube had become disconnected. What was being pumped out of my stomach was spilling all over me. It was gross, but I was relieved that it was not blood. So many odd things like that can happen. I took it in stride. I believed that God only gives challenges to those who can handle them, so there was nothing for me to worry about.

The first few nights in the hospital were restless ones. My body felt stiff, even though I had been walking up and down the halls. I felt like a child trying to walk for the first time. Although the surgery had been a success, I was still in pain, which was to be expected. I was given a painkiller every four hours. The medication helped for a while, but as soon as the four hours were up, the pain was back.

Mom stayed with me about twelve hours a day. Although I would tell her to leave early and get some rest, she would not go, and I didn't really want her to leave. Three days had passed after surgery, and I had not eaten. I was very hungry, and the loud growling noises in my stomach became a joke to everyone near me. For me, a growling stomach usually meant I had to use the bathroom, but not this time. I wanted something to eat, but it would be three or four more days before I was allowed to do so – that is, when the nasogastric and intravenous tubes were removed. The tubes had become uncomfortable. I told the nurses the tubes were a pain in the butt; they said it was refreshing to hear a patient joke about such a serious issue.

Stubborn Veins

One night my hand began to swell because of the intravenous needle. It became so bad that the needle had to be taken out of my hand and put in another part of my body. The nurse on duty took the needle out of my right hand and tried to put it in my left hand, but she could not find a suitable vein. She kept poking away, with me clutching my fist as hard as I could as the pain was becoming unbearable. After about fifteen or twenty minutes she left the room to get another nurse, who also tried unsuccessfully to find a vein.

At this point, I was full of jabs from the needles, but the nurses didn't stop there; they decided to get a doctor involved. The doctor who came in the room was young and friendly and I remember thinking how attractive he was. I was sure he was going to solve the problem, and I certainly had no objections to him putting the needle in my hand. However, despite his good looks, this doctor could not get the job done. After about an hour, and fourteen needles later, the doctor decided that the best route was to put the needle near my elbow. By this time I was sweating profusely and had a pounding headache. I remember the doctor joking, "Patients like you could have a drastic effect on the hospital budget." Of course he was referring to all the needles they wasted on me. It was a good joke and I laughed, despite the discomfort. Finally the doctor succeeded in finding a vein. It was uncomfortable, but luckily I did not have to put up with it for long, as the needle was removed the next day.

About six days after the surgery, I was finally allowed to eat. I craved something tasty, and was anxious to see what my first meal would be. It wasn't, however, what I had hoped for. Jelly and beef broth. I knew it would not satisfy my hunger, but I hoped the next day would be more satisfying. The second day was the same.

I was starving at this point and began sneaking cheezies and crackers from the drawer next to my bed when the nurses weren't looking. The cheezies, a weakness of mine since childhood, tasted delicious. I even sneaked cheezies while the intravenous was still hooked up to me. I knew this was not allowed, but I had no willpower. Fortunately, on day three the food was great. I had prayed for real food and I got it. I enjoyed a delicious breakfast, which consisted of eggs, sunny-side up, toast, and a muffin. I ate every crumb and wished for more.

Removing the Last Tube

But before I was allowed to eat solid food, the nasogastric tube had to be removed. I dreaded that day. When the nurse came into my room to advise me that the tube would be removed, I shuddered. I had been brave up to this point, but there was something about the naso-gastric tube that made me queasy, and I felt a headache coming on. The tube, extending all the way down through my stomach, had to come up the same way it went down. The only difference was that I had been asleep when the tube had gone in, but I would be awake when it was taken out.

The headache worsened. Mom went back and forth to the bathroom getting cold cloths to put on my head like she had done so many times before. The sweat was running down my face, and I was terrified at having that tube removed. My headache became so bad that it hurt to blink and then I started to cry, which made it worse. Mom thought it was a tension headache because I was so worried about the removal of the tube. Whatever it was, I don't think I had ever experienced a headache so painful before.

Waiting for the nurse to arrive made me more tense. Mom, wearing her usual brave face, sat in a chair in my room. The dreaded moment had arrived. The nurse told me it would only take a few seconds to pull out the tube – I tried hard to believe her. She looked at me with a comforting smile and asked, "Are you ready?" "As ready as I'll every be," I replied. Mom left the room. I took a deep breath. The nurse positioned me on the bed and pulled the tube. It was the most surreal feeling of all. Suddenly it was over. Granted, my nose felt like it was a foot wide and an elephant had been stuffed into it, but what a relief! Mom came back in the room with a grin on her face. She did not hear me squeal so she assumed I was fine. "Nothing to it," she said in a relieved voice.

Laughter as Therapy

Although I had several frightening experiences while I was hospitalized for bowel surgery, other times I laughed so much that it caused me physical pain. During my two-week stay in the hospital, friends, relatives, and co-workers came to visit almost every day. They always made me laugh or helped put a smile on my face. They either told me a joke or said something silly that would make me laugh so much I would practically cry in pain – with my stapled stomach, laughing was uncomfortable. In fact, it caused great discomfort, but simply being able to laugh was worth it.

One night the afternoon DJ from the Gander radio station and the news reporter from the Bay Roberts station sneaked into my room after visiting hours were over. I was surprised when they crept into my room like two young children coming home after curfew. They sat on my bed telling jokes and making me laugh (which was killing me because of the staples in my stomach); at the same time I begged them to be quiet because the nurses would come in and find them. It was like a real party. My stomach was sore from laughing so much. But I slept well that night.

A memorable, but less humorous, moment for me was when my staples were removed. I was scared, but I kept reminding myself that as soon as the staples were gone, I was another step closer to going home. The dreaded time came. A nurse was accompanied by a student nurse who would remove my staples – this was just as new to her as it was for me. Knowing she was a student made me even more nervous, but I felt relieved as soon as the process began. It was a funny, tickling feeling, but certainly not a painful one. When the staples were removed, I could finally leave the hospital.

Going Home

I walked slowly down the hall and said good-bye to the nurses. Even though I was happy to be leaving the hospital, I felt sad because I had gotten to know so many kind people. The caring way I was treated by nurses and doctors had a major impact on me. I learned firsthand the importance of a nurse. I thought nurses were a gift from Heaven, given the patience they had, tending to many sick people like me. I could see that they put up with a lot of demands from some patients – I not only witnessed it, I was a prime example. While I tried not to bother them too much, I often hit the buzzer on my pillow for one reason or another, usually because I urgently needed to use the bathroom or I wanted to go for a stroll down the hall. But I never once heard a nurse complain. They treated me like a friend. When Mom left every day after visiting hours and before she arrived each morning, I depended on the nurses to keep my spirits up, which they did just by showing they cared.

Besides my friend Sheila Collins from Hare Bay, a student nurse, who was always looking out for me, another nurse – Jane Ball – left an impression on me. Jane had an aura of optimism about her; I loved to be around her. She was the most caring and likeable nurse I had ever encountered. She always wore a smile and was very upbeat – I thought she reminded me of myself.

As Jane had experience treating patients with Crohn's disease, she could relate to my pain and frustration. Many days when I needed someone to talk to about my illness, Jane always took the time to chat with me, and she was a great listener. Often I just needed to talk, to unload my frustrations and feelings about my health. I probably sounded like a bewildered, emotional patient, but Jane listened intently. She had a keen sense of humour and she was one of the nurses who had teased me about my fancy green nightgown and robe. When I was discharged from the hospital, it was difficult to say good-bye to Jane. We exchanged the typical "I'll probably see you around sometime," but Jane and I both knew that we might never see each other again. When Sheila and I left the hospital on the day I was discharged, all I wanted to do was eat. And eat was what I did – at a pizza place that evening, with Sheila and a few friends. I knew it wasn't good for me – I had just been discharged from the hospital and I was not supposed to be eating heavy foods so soon, but I was a stubborn person that night. As a nurse and a friend, Sheila warned me not to eat too much, but despite the painful attack I had had at the Italian restaurant in Gander the previous year, I ignored her advice. None of the food I ate was healthy, except for my glass of milk. Amazingly, unlike the other incident, I did not get sick.

When I was discharged from the hospital, I was given specific instructions about my diet and I was reminded of the diet's value to my health. The doctor ordered me to stay away from certain foods (an order I was following) and to get lots of rest; I was also given instructions regarding my medications. I was advised it would be three or four months before I could return to work. That day could not come soon enough, as I wanted to get my life and job back.

I had been through quite an ordeal for the past few weeks and I really wanted to be home with my family and friends. It was a happy day for me when Dad picked me up to bring me back to Hare Bay. We had a long drive ahead of us; all I wanted was to get home without experiencing too much discomfort. I felt like someone disabled as Dad helped me into the car. I lay on the back seat all the way home. The four-hour drive felt like four days, with every little bump on the road feeling like torture. When I walked inside the trailer, I could smell Mom's delicious dinner. I had missed her cooking.

Eager to Return to Work

The next few months were boring. I lay around the trailer and did nothing; I was still weak and trying to gain my strength every day. Mom cheered me on and made sure I had plenty to eat. Friends and family visited regularly, which also made it easier to get through each day without too much worry about what lay ahead for me.

The first few weeks after surgery I did not experience much pain. I thought that the surgery had been the solution to my problems. I was feeling well, even though I was still using the bathroom frequently, even in March, almost two months after my surgery. I experienced some abdominal discomfort and found myself sitting down often because I got weak when I stood for long periods of time. I worried about it, but I didn't think it was anything too serious. Besides, I had to return to St. John's in mid-March for a check-up.

My visit with Dr. Gardiner went well. He wrote a note to my employer stating that he anticipated that I would be able to return to work by the end of April. At last, I was finally going back to work. During my months of recovery I had prepared for that day, sitting at the table in Mom's trailer with my old black tape recorder practicing reading the news. I wrote fictional news stories and recorded myself. Now I would be given a second chance to pursue my dream.

By this time, I was completely off Prednisone, the steroid responsible for my weight gain. It could not have happened soon enough, and I was finally starting to look like my normal self. My physical appearance was important to me. It had been enough that I was suffering on the inside with an ugly and chronic disease, but it was unfair that I also had to suffer the visible side effects of steroids. The drug also caused mood swings, which were completely beyond my control. Lucky for me it was in my nature to be an upbeat person, so I did a good job hiding many of my down times.

One day, during a bout of sadness, Mom and I went into a convenience store in Gambo on our way back from a doctor's appointment in Gander. As we wandered around the store, I saw a humorous wooden plaque with a picture of a duck and a caption which read: "The Secret of Success is to Stay Cool and Calm on Top and Paddle Like Hell Underneath." It made a world of sense to me, so I bought it. In an odd way, it summarized my goal of remaining hopeful that one day I would have my successful career, despite having Crohn's, as well as a happy and fulfilled life.

What Is Important

Returning to Hare Bay to recuperate made me think often about how we take things for granted, especially those things that should be most important to us, such as family, friends, and good health. My ordeal brought me closer to my family. Just as I had depended on Mom to help me when I was a young child crying out from my bedroom in pain, I depended on her now when I returned home after surgery. While I recuperated I still cried out to Mom many nights because of the pain. Even though I was a grown woman, some nights it felt like I was reliving episodes of my childhood pain and torment. My time spent in Hare Bay getting my disease under control gave me the opportunity to spend more time with Dad. We even picked out a Christmas tree together. I was 21 years old, but it was the first time that I could remember going out with Dad to cut a Christmas tree. While trying to get the Crohn's under control was not pleasurable, I also felt grateful that the experience resulted in the gift of a special bond with my parents – a rare bond between a parent and child, which, if I had not been so sick, might not have been created. The bond remains.

GERALD POOLE
RAMEA
AGE: 44

I was diagnosed eleven years ago with Crohn's disease. At first I had no idea what was wrong with me. After years of suffering with eight or nine bowel movements a day and having to be near a washroom most of the time, I finally found the answer to my problem.

My wife and I talked to other Crohn's sufferers in my home community of Ramea and I soon realized that my symptoms were almost the same as theirs. I was prescribed medication for about five years and was then told that I was in remission. One year later I was hospitalized to have 30 centimetres of my intestines removed. I came through surgery with both an ileostomy and colostomy. It was a very painful experience and something that I hope I will never have to go through again.

Although Crohn's is a painful and trying disease, I have learned that through diet and medication the disease can be controlled. The most difficult thing for me in dealing with Crohn's was trying to find the right diet – knowing what foods were going to irritate me. I have learned that if you do not take care of yourself, the disease will end your life. (My bowels ruptured just before I had surgery and I was lucky to be in a hospital at that time.)

In the early stages of my diagnosis, I was very embarrassed about having Crohn's disease and I didn't want to talk about it. Today, however, after experiencing Crohn's in the most painful way possible and learning so much about it, I am proud to say that I am comfortable discussing Crohn's disease with anyone. I now have a more active lifestyle – playing hockey, hunting, fishing, and walking, and I have more control over my body. Crohn's has also given me the strength to give up smoking for more than four years and to live a more healthy life. My coping mechanism is my determination not to let Crohn's take charge of my life and to do what I can to educate others about this very painful disease.

CHAPTER TWELVE

A Career Setback

*M*arch went by quickly, but my health was not improving as fast as I had hoped. I was still experiencing pain and made frequent trips to the bathroom; it became clear that I could not return to work in April. I was really frustrated; it didn't seem like I would ever be able to get on with my life. I was a young woman fighting a horrible disease, and this setback didn't seem fair. What if I stayed off work too long and lost my job? I was now afraid that I would never be able to go back to work at the radio station in Gander. However, as upsetting as it was, my health had to come first and I needed to deal with this situation the best way I could. Even so, I struggled to keep a positive attitude.

I was advised that I would have to go on long-term disability. My employer had paid me while I was on short-term sick leave, but now I would be paid by the insurance company. I completed all the necessary steps to qualify for long-term disability benefits. My doctor wrote a letter to the radio station advising them of my medical condition. It felt so final, and I was depressed. I could not believe that a young woman in her early twenties was now about to go on long-term disability. It was as if my career had ended even before it began. How could this happen? This had to be a horrible dream and I would wake up soon, I thought.

The Need to Get Away

One day after my long-term disability was sorted out, I sat alone in Mom's trailer and decided that I needed to get away from everything and everyone for a while. I wanted to forget that I had Crohn's and how this disease had taken away my job and now controlled my life. Every day I was reminded of my chronic illness. I desperately needed a change of pace; I wanted to get away and have fun.

I decided to go on a trip. I had received an invitation from my cousin in Ontario who was getting married in April. I had always wanted to visit her. My sister Dana and Aunt Glenda were going, and I thought it would do me good to be around family that I had not seen for such a long time. My brother Dirk, whom I had not seen in a while, would also be there.

While I was excited about going to Ontario, I kept wondering if I was healthy enough to take the trip. What if I had an attack on the plane? What if I became seriously ill at the wedding? I had mixed feelings. The next day I received Dr. Hewitt's opinion on travelling. I explained to him that not only did I want to be part of my cousin's special day, but I also needed to do something that would help me feel like a normal person again. Dr. Hewitt did not have any major concerns and thought it was a good idea. I was excited, and it was refreshing to hear something positive.

My family in Ontario were looking forward to seeing me, especially after all my health problems. My Aunt Beulah, for whom I am named (my middle name is Beulah), was elated that I was coming to Ontario. I had never forgotten the day she phoned me when I was rushed to the hospital in Gander; she told me then that she would pray for me every day until I was well again. It was good to know that people were praying for me.

The hour-long drive to the Gander airport was without incident – no stomach ache and no need to stop along the way to use the bathroom. I had a great feeling about this trip and a sense of excitement that I had not felt in a very long time. I would soon be in the magnificent city of Toronto, where so many Newfoundlanders and Labradorians have flocked over the years. The plane trip was exhausting, however, as I tired easily.

When we arrived at the church the following day, I was greeted by old friends and family that I had not seen in a long time, who commented on how well I looked, considering my ordeal with Crohn's disease. There were many compliments, but I still felt paranoid about my looks. My face was still rounded from steroid use, even though I no longer took them. My brother Dirk was happy to see me and he did not care what my face looked like. Spending time with him made the trip to Ontario even more worthwhile.

I did find myself from time to time explaining Crohn's disease. I didn't mind talking about it, but I could sense that others weren't quite as comfortable talking about the disease as I was. While Crohn's disease was becoming more common, I sensed that some people didn't think it was appropriate to talk about this disease in public. However, my immediate family and friends were interested, so I just kept on talking. I was amazed at how little people knew about Crohn's.

I looked forward to going home, probably because I felt secure around Mom and Dad. Some people like to be alone when they aren't feeling well. I was the opposite; I wanted to be around friends and family. I think I needed to be near family and friends because of all of the unknowns associated with Crohn's disease. Being around familiar people helped take my mind off my illness.

When I returned to Hare Bay I realized that the trip had indeed been good therapy – it felt good to be part of such a positive and joyful occasion. While I did think about the possibility of getting sick while I was away, I tried not to let it bother me. Other than occasional abdominal pains and frequent trips to the bathroom, which were typical for me, my trip went well.

Coping, One Step at a Time

At home, the disease continued to be unpredictable, which was most frustrating. I had good days where I felt like I could take on the world, but then I'd have days when I was utterly miserable as a result of weakness and anxiety over my predicament.

Soon it was May and the snow had almost disappeared. With summer approaching, my spirits began to lift. My condition continued to be monitored by my doctor. I started to feel bored, which I took as a sign that I was getting better. The next holiday was Victoria Day – a long weekend that I had always looked forward to. I wanted to go camping with my friends, but I wasn't sure if I was ready to rough it in the woods, given my frequent trips to the bathroom and the fact that I was no longer a normal, healthy person. But getting out in the fresh air also appealed to me. Now that I had Crohn's disease there were many new considerations, and I couldn't just simply go like before.

Some friends and I decided to stay at a cabin at Spruce Grove

Resort near Square Pond Provincial Park. It was only about a half-hour drive from Hare Bay. Staying in a cabin rather than in a tent was much more comfortable for me. Camping in the cool weather probably would not have been a prudent choice. Other than the fact that I was probably the first to go to bed at night because I was tired, I felt normal during the entire holiday weekend. We laughed and had fun.

After this holiday, I started to go out more frequently, to movies and to local night clubs from time to time with my friends. Because of my rounded face and extra weight resulting from fluid retention and increased appetite, it took time to get over my paranoia of being in a public place. Although the doctors had told me that these visible side effects of Prednisone were reversible, the process was taking too long.

The Power of Milk

I often did not drink alcohol when I was at a night club because it sometimes hurt my stomach; I did not want to risk the pain. I was also on medications, which meant that I was not allowed to drink alcohol. For a while, I drank only white milk when I was out with my friends. Along with pineapple juice, milk did not hurt my stomach, which was odd in one sense because many IBD sufferers are lactose intolerant. I loved milk; it did not hurt me, but I needed ice in it.

One night I asked a bartender for a glass of milk with ice. I'll never forget the strange look on his face when he asked me what I would like in my milk. I told him I wanted ice. He shook his head in amazement because I was not drinking alcohol. I thought it was funny, but I was also intrigued by his reaction to my request for a glass of milk. Did he think I was strange for wanting to drink milk at a bar? Did he think that people should only drink alcohol in a bar? If so, then I figured the bartender was not the only one who thought it was strange to see someone drinking milk in a bar. While I was drinking my milk one evening, a guy came over to talk to me. I didn't know him, but he obviously wanted to get to know me. I thought to myself, hopefully, that perhaps I didn't look too bad after all, despite my balloon-shaped face. He asked me what I was drinking, presumably because he was going to buy me a drink. I told him I was drinking milk. He did not believe me. He said, "You're joking, right?" After what turned into a short, meaningless discussion about what I was drinking, he looked at me and said, "I don't mean to sound bold, but are you pregnant or something?" I started to laugh and almost spit milk in his face. I thought this guy was a real loser. After realizing what he had said, he apologized and stressed that he had not meant to hurt my feelings or speak out of line.

I could not stop laughing. I thought it was amazing how people assume that everyone in a bar is drinking alcohol. The guy left the bar area where my friends and I were standing; drinking milk probably wasn't sexy enough for him. Maybe I should have ventured into a deep conversation about IBD and told him I had Crohn's disease and how drinking alcohol was bad for my bowels, and how some days I would have to go to the bathroom about a dozen times. I could only imagine his reaction.

CHAPTER THIRTEEN

A Gradual Return to Work

*I*t was June 5, 1988 – my birthday. I was now 22 years old. I had started walking and exercising and I was feeling good about myself, better than I had felt in the past year or so. I was ready and eager to get back to work, at least on a temporary basis. In late June my doctor decided I could go back into the workforce. It was a big step for me – another sign of a return to normalcy. I would first go back on a trial basis.

The doctor, however, felt I was not prepared or ready to return to work under the same circumstances as before. Being the only newsperson at the radio station often meant long hours and hectic days; this is fine for a healthy person, but it would not be wise for me to return immediately to such a routine. In the past, there were many days when I had worked from 5:45 a.m. to 2:00 p.m., and again in the evening to cover a meeting or conference. I knew it would take time to get back into this routine, but I was eager to work full time. I needed to prove to myself and to my family, friends, and co-workers that despite having Crohn's I could still live a fairly normal life and have a career.

I would work regular eight-hour days at the radio station for a few months to see how I managed. The plan was to gradually build up my strength and ease myself back into what had been a typical day at work. I was satisfied with the plan, and anxious to get moving.

Additional Challenges

But, it wasn't so simple. Another hurdle was put in front of me. During my time on sick leave, the company that owned the radio station had undergone changes, including lay-offs. One of the cutbacks was the news position in Gander – my position. I was technically without a job. I did, however, have seniority over some of the other workers, so there would be a job available for me, but not in Gander. I would have to move to another radio station. I was discouraged. I had enough to deal with already; I did not need this extra worry or stress. Why was I having so much bad luck?, I asked myself.

Since I was only back to work on a trial basis, I had to concentrate on getting back into a normal work routine. I knew it would not be easy. I would have to work around my illness while also trying to prove to myself and my boss that I was still able to do my job efficiently and professionally. One of my biggest worries was the unpredictability of another attack. The uncertainty of another flare-up and how long it could last was particularly tormenting. I had horrible thoughts about covering a news conference, and, right in the middle of the event, needing to rush off to the bathroom, or, even worse, I would not make it to the bathroom on time. I could never handle that.

While I was excited about returning to work, I felt uneasy about the changes in the company. I tried to brush it off, and I gradually moved myself back into a work routine. But the diarrhea persisted. Some days I used the bathroom ten or twelve times. The doctor gave me various medications to control the diarrhea – Questran, Imodium, and Lomotil. It seemed that each medication worked for a short period of time. Lomotil was the most effective of the three drugs and I stayed on it for several years.

I spent considerable time in the small bathroom at CFYQ radio station. It had a small window, and many times I tried to keep the window open, to vent the unpleasant smell, just in case someone came in immediately behind me. I always carried matches with me – they were perfect to mask the smell. Some days I cried in embarrassment and other days I was in the bathroom with the window open, lighting matches, and laughing to myself, thinking how in the name of God am I going to live life like this. I tried to find humour in such awkward situations.

I feared that I would be reading the news one day and all of a sudden have to use the bathroom or that I would experience abdominal pain like I had so many times before, which caused me to hide in my office at work so that nobody could see me cry in pain. What I feared most was the unknown; I feared a major attack and having to leave work again. I thought that no company would tolerate such behaviour.

The pessimism was eating away at me, but I knew I had to pull myself together and make this return to work a success. I wanted both my job and my health, and I had to prove that I could overcome the challenges. I felt I was being given a second chance so I wanted to show everyone who knew me that I was determined to get well and do the best I could in all things, no matter where my career path took me.

The time had come to make a decision about where I would work. What would be best for me now that I was easing myself back into my news reporter's job? I would have to pick up where I left off a year earlier. The thought of having to leave Gander and move to another town to work with different people at a different radio station wasn't welcomed by me or my doctor. It would be stressful for a healthy individual to be uprooted from his/her home and to start over in another town. But it would be even more difficult for someone who was battling a chronic illness like Crohn's to ease back into the workforce.

My doctor was in Gander and my family and friends were nearby. I needed my doctor, family, and friends near me as they played a role in my efforts to learn how to live with Crohn's disease, especially at this early stage. I especially wanted to be near Dr. Hewitt; I couldn't imagine being under another doctor's care.

I was also getting established in Gander as a reporter, trying to develop working relationships and proving myself to the community. I was young, but I believed I had potential, and I wanted to stay in Gander to gain the experience I hoped would open career doors. Above all, I was just plain scared: change is difficult for any individual. Unfortunately, although I had many reasons to stay in Gander, there was one overriding reason why I could not – there was no job there for me.

After reviewing my options and having further discussions with my doctor and a representative of the union at work, a decision was finally reached with the company. I would return to the Gander radio station on a six-month trial basis, but my job duties would change. During this period, I would work with the secretary and do administrative-type work, as well as some in-house news, but I would not cover community news events: I was not ready, health-wise, for such a high-paced activity, and, due to the lay-offs, there was no longer a news position at the Gander station.

I felt comfortable that the trial arrangement would allow me to ease back into work – it would be a test to determine if I was capable of doing my job like before. After the trial period, a decision would be made regarding which radio station I would be transferred to – that is, if I was healthy and reliable enough to work in a news department again.

Happier Days

I had been waiting for what seemed like forever to return to work, and I felt it was now within my reach. I still had to go through much red tape before I could officially return to work. In October, I was finally given the go-ahead to return to work after the Thanksgiving Day weekend. I was ecstatic! More than ten months before I had been so sick that I thought I would never return to radio work. Now, I was starting over. It was appropriate to be thankful on this Thanksgiving Day.

I honestly believed that all those prayers that my family prayed for me, especially my Aunt Beulah's daily prayer and my Nan Collins's prayers, were effective. Nan always worried about me, especially when I was attending college in Stephenville. She constantly talked about how sick I was and that she could not imagine how I managed to deal with my illness on my own. After I graduated, Nan's favourite words to me were, "I don't know how you did it all the way over there by yourself. You were so sick." I often think of these words, and her concern for my well-being.

When I received permission to return to work, I wanted to shout it out to the world. I was anxious to share the good news with my family, friends, and even strangers. I think my parents were more relieved and thankful than I was. It had been a trying year for them, but they never gave up on me or their belief that I would soon be back in the workforce.

I could not sleep the night before my return to work. My mind was full of possible scenarios of what was waiting for me. My alarm went off at 7:00 a.m. I listened to the radio for a few minutes before I got out of bed. This was it. I decided to wear a new dress that I had recently bought, thinking that this day would soon arrive. I was nervous. It seemed like forever since I last worked. I walked with great pride into the radio station the first morning after being off for almost a year. I gently sat in my old chair in the newsroom office; it felt like home.

That first day was routine. I got reacquainted with my co-workers, especially the secretary, with whom I would be working, and refamiliarized myself with the environment. As I would be doing in-house news under the new arrangement, I was looking forward to going through my old files and digging out some contacts in order to get up to date on the latest happenings in and around Gander.

I used the bathroom often that first day. I guess it was a combination of nerves and my medical condition. By the end of the day, the constant trips to the bathroom had left me a little weak. I felt embarrassed leaving the office so much, but after a few weeks I got over it. There was no need for me to feel embarrassed or ashamed; I had a serious illness and the staff knew it. A month passed and I was doing well at work, and my health was holding its own. I felt confident that things would continue to improve for me if I continued to work hard and take care of myself.

Creating IBD Awareness

I became more involved in the Gander chapter of the Canadian Foundation for Ileitis and Colitis. November was a public awareness month across Canada and CFIC's biggest fundraiser was underway – its annual Christmas cake sale. The radio station helped the Gander chapter in its fundraising efforts by giving free air time for public service announcements and promoting CFIC's Christmas cake sale. I was busy with my volunteer activities, and after working all day at the station, I often felt exhausted. I had to stay off work one day in November as I felt especially weak and experienced some pain in my belly. It was nothing serious; it was just my body telling me to slow down.

In November, as part of Crohn's and Colitis Awareness Month, I received a phone call from CBC Radio in Gander. They wanted to interview me about my experience with Crohn's disease. I was pleased to be asked to talk about IBD as I felt it was important to use every opportunity to speak publicly about this chronic illness. I wanted to educate people about IBD and this was the first time that I would go public with my story. When CBC asked me to do the interview, my thoughts went to others who were going through what I had experienced for such a long time. I wanted to use the media interview as a way to reach out to sufferers of IBD and assure them they were not alone.

The president of the Gander chapter of the CFIC, Mary Cheeseman, was also invited to participate in the interview. Mary and I had been working together closely since my involvement in CFIC. Although our chapter was small, the executive was a great team and I was proud to be the vice-president – a position I took seriously. The interview went well. We thanked the CBC for giving us the opportunity to talk about Crohn's disease and colitis, and to advise people of a support group in the Gander area. We also extended an invitation to the public to take part in our chapter meetings.

At my first meeting at the Gander chapter of the CFIC I had felt so out of place; I wanted to get out of the room as fast as I could. But when people started talking about their experiences with IBD, I immediately felt a connection with them. Their stories were like mine, and it was as if they were telling mine for me. I could relate to them, and I no longer regarded these people as strangers. Above all, I realized that I was not alone. Listening to people from all walks of life share their stories during chapter meetings made a difference in my attitude towards IBD, which many sufferers are afraid to talk about publicly. At the end of the first meeting, I felt empowered to educate people about IBD, and to be a support system for sufferers needing someone to talk to about their frustrations. I realized that IBD sufferers are indeed ordinary people who have been handed a difficult and painful challenge and they should never be ashamed of having this disease or be embarrassed to talk about it.

My involvement in CFIC also strengthened my ability to cope with Crohn's, and I eagerly encouraged others to get involved in what

I considered a worthy cause. My family and friends supported our fundraising events. Many of them had observed the effects of my disease and they understood the importance of creating an awareness about the illness and raising funds for IBD research. My family and friends wished that a cure could be found for Crohn's disease as much as I did.

BEVERLY SWACKHAMER
BARENEED
AGE: 40

My experience with Crohn's disease has been a long and painful one. I was diagnosed when I was nineteen. I have been fighting the disease ever since. Over half my life has been spent in a battle with a disease that nobody can tell me why I have it, or how to get rid of it.

The downside of this illness has been being in pain almost all the time – painful tests, awful medications, long hospital stays, and three bowel surgeries. But, some positive things have come from having Crohn's disease. I have become involved with a great group of people who are all working hard to raise money for research into finding a cure for Crohn's. I have developed strong bonds with other Crohn's sufferers in Newfoundland and Labrador, as well as with those whose family members suffer from Crohn's. I have also had the privilege of meeting people from across Canada who have this horrible disease.

Eight years after my second surgery I gave birth to my first daughter, Madelyn. Two years later, I gave birth to Christina. They were miracles! I was told that because of my illness I would never have children. They are truly gifts from God. I keep up my determination in fundraising for the Crohn's and Colitis Foundation of Canada because of them now. I'm not looking for a cure for myself. I'm trying to help ensure that if my children get this disease there will be a cure available immediately. I don't want them to go through what I've been through.

Living with Crohn's disease has been really hard, but it has also given me a chance to help others, which I enjoy very much. I have talked to people who were newly diagnosed. I have talked to people before and after surgery. I have tried to give people a little hope that they will feel normal again one day. Knowing that I have helped people cope with this illness makes me feel a little better for having to suffer through it.

I hope that I will live long enough to see the day when a cure for Crohn's is found. It would be a great ending to a long and tiring battle.

CHAPTER FOURTEEN

Other Consequences of Crohn's

*N*ovember went by quickly, and the Christmas season was just around the corner. Everything was going well except I could not get rid of the pressure and tightness in my stomach and abdominal area. The pain was not as frequent as before, but it was persistent. It was something I now simply accepted, and I coped as well as I could. I was determined not to let the pain ruin my holidays. One thing was certain, I felt much better than I had the previous Christmas.

In December, along with an occasional night disturbed by abdominal aches, I started to experience intense pain in my joints, specifically my wrists and ankles. It kept me awake at night, with the pain usually coming in spurts. The symptoms lasted for two or three nights and then didn't come back for another week or so. I put off going to the doctor, however, because I didn't want something else to worry about.

A dose of laughter always got me through the rough times, but, being human, at times I found it hard to keep a smile on my face as the pain worsened. I tried hard not to let people see that I wasn't feeling well, as I wanted everybody to see a normal, happy-go-lucky woman, free of pain. I could not fool everyone, though, especially Mom.

I spent Christmas Day in Hare Bay. Much of the holiday was spent in bed because of my aching joints, with my wrists and ankles feeling like they were on fire. Some nights the pain was so bad that I paced the floor in Mom's trailer for hours, praying for the aching to end. I eventually told Dr. Hewitt about it early in January. He explained that it is not uncommon for people with IBD to suffer from joint pain and experience arthritis-like conditions. He did say, however, that joint pain doesn't usually occur until after someone has had the disease for several years. He thought it was unusual that I was experiencing joint pain so soon after my diagnosis. Whether it was considered unusual or not, the pain was real and it kept me awake at night. However, since the aching wasn't constant, my doctor decided not to prescribe more medication. Instead, my situation would be monitored to see how I felt in a few weeks. I had had more than my share of drugs – having to take more medication was definitely not appealing.

I continued to learn about Crohn's disease. Even though I had read all of the information I could get on IBD, there was so much more to learn. It is a frustrating and unpredictable disease – just when you think you know all about the illness and everything is under control, something else pops up. Everything about IBD perplexed me.

I promised myself that I would do everything I could to make 1989 a good year. I kept busy at work and wrote more local news stories. Eventually, I covered some Gander Town Council meetings, which were held every second Wednesday. It felt great walking into the council chambers again. The other media and councillors welcomed me back; it was encouraging that they hadn't forgotten me. I was proud to be back. I felt as though my career was getting back on track and I prayed that this was the beginning of a road to a brighter future.

The first few months of 1989 were great. I was feeling healthy and the aching in my wrists and ankles had eased. As things were looking up for me, I decided to make myself busier. There was some extra energy brewing and I wasn't about to let it go to waste. I always loved to keep busy; my health issues hadn't changed that about me.

I decided that I would do some work outside the radio station – maybe some freelancing. I had done some freelance work in the past for such publications as *The Newfoundland Herald*. I loved writing, especially lifestyles stories, and, with the permission of the radio station, I decided to do some freelance work for *The Herald*. My physical state may not have been one hundred percent, but my mind was fine. I wanted to keep active and continue to gain exposure as a writer or reporter whenever and wherever possible. I also wanted to make some extra money, as the wages of community radio reporters were typically low.

Utilizing my extra energy did not end at writing for *The Herald*. I wanted to do more, so I became involved with Gander's local TV channel, Channel 9. I did several documentaries on the 1985 Arrow Air crash in Gander and later reported on Town Council meetings for Channel 9. TV work was exciting and I gained valuable experience. Most days, I felt like a bird soaring high in the sky where nothing could bring me down from the feeling of being so free and happy. Maybe one day I would become a well-known TV news anchor. I always believed that no dream was too big. I also became more physically active. I jogged and walked in the evenings – anything that kept me fit and made me feel good about myself was on my list of priorities. I welcomed the days when my life felt like it was moving forward the way I had hoped, but I could not escape those few unpredictable days when I felt like a truck had run over me. It was as if I was always yanked back by some mysterious power as a reminder that I had Crohn's disease and I wasn't allowed to be pain-free every day. It was annoying, but I kept plugging along and, when I was feeling good, I took advantage of every minute. I learned how to focus on today and not worry about what tomorrow would bring. I was determined to win this fight, one battle at a time.

I continued my involvement in the Gander chapter of CFIC as vice-president. March was the Strike out Ileitis and Colitis Campaign, a national fundraiser involving the Toronto Blue Jays and Montreal Expos. These two Canadian baseball teams wanted to help the CFIC raise money and create an awareness of IBD. People donated money for every strike-out acquired by the pitching staff of either the Blue Jays or the Expos at the end of the baseball season. The radio station helped promote this exciting event. I was once again pleased by the station's support of the CFIC.

In April I was just one month away from deciding which radio station I would work at, and my time in Gander would soon become part of my past. The six-month work agreement would be re-evaluated at the end of May, and I would have to leave Gander if I wanted a job. My options: Grand Falls or St. John's.

I knew I was ready to return to a full-time radio reporter's job. I wanted to work in a news department, like my old job two years earlier. But I wanted to be healthy and return to work without worrying about having to go on sick leave again.

The company's news director, Brendan McCarthy, who was based in St. John's, suggested that I move to St. John's to work in the newsroom. He thought it would be a good career move for me. Even at decision time, I was hoping that I would not have to work anywhere else but Gander. I was afraid of leaving my family, my doctor, and my friends. Besides my health concerns, I also feared living alone in a big city where I did not know anyone. It was similar to the feeling I had the day I boarded the CN bus in 1984 to attend college in Stephenville. What if I became sick in the middle of the night in St. John's? Who would I call?

I acknowledged that the radio station in St. John's was where the news happened. The provincial news was written in St. John's and then provided to the smaller stations, such as the one in Gander. I wondered about the potential stress associated with working at such a large radio station where the pace would be faster and more eyes would be focused on me and my performance. Although the influence of stress in Crohn's disease is being debated in the scientific community, I was almost convinced that taking on more responsibilities in a larger radio station would cause a flare-up of Crohn's.

Fearing Change

My thinking was erratic. My emotions were making me sick. For a while, I came up with every possible reason why I should not move to St. John's, when I knew I should be focusing on the positive aspects of such a move. I needed a reminder of my glass-is-half-full-not-half-empty attitude. It was time for me to have an open mind and view change as an opportunity.

A few days later, after I had another check-up with my family doctor and after a long talk with the general manager of the Q-Radio network in St. John's, I decided to speak to the news director again about the position. I wanted more information on the type of work I would be doing, the hours of work, who I would be working with, and so on.

The general manager told me it was fine to be scared, but he encouraged me. He had listened to some of my news reports and felt I had the potential to advance in radio if I put my mind to it. For me, however, the main issue wasn't about my desire to gain the experience and hopefully advance my career, it was completely about my health. All of a sudden I was still scared of going back to work full-time in a new and fast-paced environment because it could be detrimental to my health.

Everyone I spoke with said that I should grasp this opportunity – to them, I was fortunate to be given the chance to build my career. The general manager reminded me that if my health didn't deteriorate then there was no reason why I could not have the career I had always dreamed of. My telephone conversation with him made me see things in a different perspective. I was elated that he saw my potential, but I was still confused.

I also thought about how I did not want to let my parents down by not pursing a new career opportunity and moving on with my life. I felt like I had been a burden on them for the past few years, especially on Mom, so if I moved to St. John's it would be a relief for them as it would show that the pieces of my life that had been torn apart by Crohn's were finally being put back together. In their comforting way, my parents pointed out that in St. John's I would be closer to my bowel specialist, thus avoiding those long bus trips for my check-ups.

Even with these words of encouragement, I wasn't quite ready to make up my mind just yet. I needed some time to clear my head. I decided that when I went to St. John's for my appointment with Dr. Higgins on May 19 I would meet with Brendan McCarthy. While nothing was official, I really didn't have a choice but to move to St. John's if I wanted to keep my job.

The bus ride to St. John's was long and boring – too much time to think. I realized, however, that Mom and Dad were right about the long trips to have my check-ups. Not having to do that anymore would be a relief.

Cecil Haire, who also worked in the newsroom at the Q-Radio and KIXX FM network in St. John's, met me at the bus terminal. I had not seen Cecil since he visited me in the hospital in St. John's when I had my bowel re-section. We discussed my health and work over supper. Like me, Cecil was an upbeat person and our discussion improved my confidence. He felt I would be better off in St. John's, from both a health and career perspective. I agreed, but my health concerns always tipped the scale. I still struggled with the mindset that my illness narrowed my focus.

My health was improving so I was anticipating a good check-up with Dr. Higgins, and, therefore, I was eager to meet with him again. I was not feeling as relaxed, though, about my pending meeting with Brendan to discuss my new job; I was nervous.

This trip to St. John's proved to be a transition in my life. Arriving in St. John's and meeting co-workers and friends showed that I could resume a normal life. On my first night in the city, we decided to go out on the town and visit George Street. It was a big deal for me considering the emotional time I had been having with the changes taking place in my life in order to adapt to a new life with a bowel disease. I told the story about the guy at the bar in Gander who had given me a difficult time about drinking milk. I joked that maybe I should stick to drinking milk to see what reaction I'd get from people.

It was not a late night for me as I had an appointment with Dr. Higgins the next day, but socializing and meeting new people made me feel alive again. I realized that I could still have fun, even with Crohn's disease. It was clear that the night life in St. John's – a place I could soon call home – was exciting. But, for me, just living in a large city would be a learning experience in itself. I could add that to my list of reasons why St. John's would be a great place to live. The extent of the night life in a small community like Hare Bay was the Royal Canadian Legion, Branch 69. Yes, the Legion was the place to be in Hare Bay on a Saturday night. But, it was not George Street in downtown St. John's.

CHAPTER FIFTEEN

My Second Chance at a Career

When I walked into Dr. Higgins's office on May 19, I thought I must be wearing three heads by the way he looked at me. "Are you the same girl I saw three months ago?," he asked. I certainly did not expect this question. I looked at him in amazement and asked what he meant. He told me he couldn't get over how healthy I looked and how upbeat I appeared. "It's not what's on the outside that counts, it's what's on the inside that matters," I replied jokingly. I had to agree with him, though, I did look and feel better. Looking in the mirror no longer angered me; I liked what I saw.

Dr. Higgins was pleased with the improvement in my health and he gave me his blessing to return to full-time work. He told me to keep smiling and that if I took good care of myself everything would be fine. Dr. Higgins was a compassionate doctor and I was lucky to be in his care. My next appointment would be in six months. Even though my health had improved, Dr. Higgins still felt I needed to be monitored, at least for now, to ensure that the disease remained under control.

When I walked out of Dr. Higgins's office that morning, I felt as though I was about to start a new life – a feeling that was becoming more common for me. I had a huge grin on my face as I said good-bye to the receptionists, to whom I was no stranger. There was no pain in my stomach that day, just butterflies from the excitement of knowing that I could now move on to the next chapter in my life.

My next stop was to meet with Brendan McCarthy at the radio station. I had only met Brendan in person once before, but from our telephone conversations I sensed he was a pleasant man, and he was well respected at the station. On my way to meet with Brendan I thought about our first encounter, when I was discharged from the Grace General Hospital following my surgery. I had dropped by the station with Rodney Etheridge for a few minutes to meet some of the staff. I was a ghastly sight that day: I was bent over because standing up straight after surgery felt like my stomach was ripping open, and I walked slowly. I remembered Brendan's display of genuine compassion and concern. He would see a different woman now – probably wouldn't even recognize me because I no longer looked like a sick, weak woman.

Brendan and I had a long chat in his office, which faced a busy Duckworth Street. Looking out the window, I noted the heavy traffic outside of his office, and I was amazed at how close the vehicles were to the building. Life in St. John's would certainly be at a faster pace than either Gander or Hare Bay. Brendan explained that the job waiting for me would see me work early morning hours on the KIXX FM Country station from 5:30 a.m. to 8:45 a.m. doing on-air traffic reports and weather information with the morning show announcer. I would be on the air every fifteen minutes. After 9:00 a.m. I would read the hourly news on the Q-93 AM station until 1:00 p.m. Brendan thought this job would be a perfect fit for me, considering my health. I would not have to be out reporting in the field, so I did not have to worry about my health in the sense of having to be on the go all the time.

Although I did not have to worry about it at the time, I had a recurring fear of having to go to the bathroom in the middle of a press conference with a room full of people. Although I joked with Brendan about it, and we made light of the situation, Brendan also understood my underlying concern and fear, given that this disease was still new to me, and still a mystery to many people. He also pointed out that the management team was also aware of my medical condition and would understand if I became sick. There were thirteen people working in the newsroom, so there would always be somebody to fill in if I became sick. This was different from the Gander station where only one person worked in the newsroom, which meant that when I became sick there was no one to replace me, and in many instances the morning DJ had to read the news.

Brendan made the job sound exciting, and told me that the company wanted a friendly female voice on the air. They felt that because of my upbeat personality I would be good for the job. The compliment meant a great deal to me, especially given the battle I had had with my self-esteem when I was on Prednisone. In a relaxed tone, Brendan convinced me that this was a great opportunity. I jokingly told Brendan he was an effective salesman. I'd be crazy not to take the job, I thought.

I made my decision: I would move to St. John's and start work the following week. The joy I felt about my new job was overwhelming. I had so much to do to prepare for the move. The only thing I dreaded was saying good-bye to my family and friends in Hare Bay and Gander. But they were just as excited as I was about the new job.

I found a one-bedroom apartment downtown, close to work. The Sunday night before my first day on the job was a restless one. Every attempt to fall asleep failed. My alarm went off at 4:30 a.m. and I walked to work that morning. I would spend the first week shadowing Cecil Haire, who was doing the job on KIXX FM that I was about to do. It did not take me long to catch on. Much of what I had to do was familiar, as I had carried out similar duties at the Gander station. My stomach was tied up in knots, not from my health condition, but from the anticipation. I was lucky I already knew many of my co-workers. I was most comforted knowing that Rodney and Cecil would be around to lend support. They had always been there to assist me when I travelled to St. John's for doctor's appointments, and knowing I had that kind of support from colleagues made me feel better about a new life in St. John's.

I was confident I would do well in this new job. The morning show host and I connected immediately. It took a few days to get into a routine, but everything fell into place. I loved my job, and life was finally returning to normal.

A Supportive Work Environment

My co-workers were helpful and understanding. I often left the newsroom to use the bathroom and sometimes I felt embarrassed about it. But they treated me no differently than anyone else, despite the paranoia I often felt. "Excuse me," was my famous saying, as I dashed off to the bathroom. Thank goodness there were fewer women working at the station in the morning than men – there were times when I just could not wait. I often remembered the conversations I had with other Crohn's sufferers during CFIC meetings in Gander when we didn't mince our words about diarrhea. So many times we used the phrase, "when you got to go, you got to go"! We always laughed when we said it, but it had a serious meaning for us, which came true for me so many times at work. Unlike most healthy people, IBD sufferers cannot *hold it.*

Eventually, my having to use the bathroom so often became a joke at work. All the guys, especially the sports editor, Craig Jackson, teased me about it. It did not bother me after a while because my co-workers were only trying to make me feel at ease about my situation. The best part was that I would always make sure that I had a good come-back for them! The laughter helped me forget about the pain and the discomfort. It was still torture at times, but I tried to keep my promise to myself not to complain about my health. I was determined to make my return to work a positive experience. I wanted my co-workers to view me as a talented individual who wanted to bring value to the radio station. I did not want to be labelled as just a worker who was always sick.

The arrival of summer meant softball season. The radio station participated in the media softball league, and since I enjoyed watching the sport, I was also eager to play. I was lucky to be living a fairly normal life and could take part in such activities. On frustrating days, I reminded myself that my challenges were minimal compared to some people's. I could play softball, while there were others who could not walk.

Connecting with IBD Sufferers

Besides focusing on learning and improving my skills at work, volunteering for the CFIC remained an important part of my life. Shortly after I arrived in St. John's I received a phone call from Joan Bessey, the president of the St. John's chapter. Joan, who also suffered from Crohn's, wanted me to get involved in her chapter. We talked about the need to improve awareness of the disease. Our first meeting was in a food court in downtown St. John's. People all around us were eating lunch while we talked about bowel disease – the contrast was funny, and we couldn't stop laughing. Talking about bowels was no big deal to us but, to some people, it is considered dirty and disgusting. It seemed that Crohn's sufferers have an odd sense of humour. Joan and I believed in the power of laughter. Soon after, I met Dianne Janes, another CFIC volunteer and Crohn's sufferer, with whom I also developed a bond. The three of us became an effective team, and proud of our cause.

I respected Joan and Dianne for their dedication to volunteerism and their sincerity about helping to find a cure for IBD. They became more than fellow volunteers; they became friends. My involvement with the CFIC in St. John's and the special people I met brought a new meaning and joy to my life. I felt as if I was making a difference in this world. Like the warm feeling I got from having my friends and family by my side at the hospital, my work with the CFIC made me happy. It also became more evident to me and to others that the happier I felt, the healthier I became.

ROXANNE WHITE
CURLING
AGE: 41

After years of gut-wrenching and all-over body pain, it took only a moment in time when my soul felt crushed and I could not handle it any longer. I recall that last night of fighting, without pain medication, an unbearable pain until the early morning. Fortunately, a doctor making his rounds, looked at me and said, "prep her for surgery now."

Although this was the third surgery, it was the one that diagnosed me as having Crohn's disease, which resulted in the removal of two feet of my bowel. It was May 1990 and I was 26 years old. When I first heard of the disease, it sounded so foreign and yet I felt like I knew this disease so well. I was actually elated because now there would be no more invasive procedures, no more medication, no more of not knowing what was wrong with me. My own doctor told me that there was nothing wrong with me, and the pain was in my head. In my heart I believe that the doctor who saved my life was meant to be there that morning. Shortly after the diagnosis I had to have a complete hysterectomy because Crohn's had infected most of my mid-section.

Regardless of what this disease robbed – time away from my son, family, friends, and opportunities – I met many great people through support groups, including other people afflicted with the disease. I am now involved with the Crohn's and Colitis Foundation of Canada and committed to our mission: to find a cure. Today, I am not on any medications, I have stayed out of the hospital since my last surgery in 1990. I am grateful that I have more good days than bad.

I thank God, my mother, family, and friends for getting me through my suffering. Every day I live with Crohn's disease, but every day Crohn's disease does not live with me. I pray that a cure will be found soon.

CHAPTER SIXTEEN

Crohn's and My Career: Continuous Learning

A few months after my arrival in St. John's, my Crohn's was still active, but, overall, I was coping well and enjoying my life and my career. The summer of 1989 ended; the softball season was over and there were no injuries. I did not get a home run, but there was always next year. My work at Q-93 AM - KIXX FM was becoming more exciting. The company decided that I would do the morning traffic reports out on the road, instead of in the studio. I would drive the company's new vehicle. I was thrilled; not only would that mean more publicity for the company, specifically for KIXX FM station, the station I would be doing the reports for, the additional exposure would also benefit my future career.

For the first time, I would be driving in St. John's. I was nervous, and being nervous made me use the bathroom, but it didn't take long for me to calm down, and soon I was having a grand time. Our morning show was called the KIXX Breakfast Mix with Brian O'Connell and Sonia Glover. Brian and I were a great match, and every morning was full of laughter. At first, I didn't have a clue what street I was on when Brian asked me on the air. He knew that I didn't know where I was and he was having fun with it – we had a ball. This was an exciting and rewarding time in my career, and I felt triumphant. I was young and proud of how far I had come in such a short time. Working with Brian on the morning show helped me grow personally and professionally, and I decided that there was no way I was going to let my health limit my career. Now, I thought, it was impossible for any illness to bring me down from this high I was experiencing.

I also had a new family doctor, Dr. Sean Conroy. He was both friendly and thorough, which were important factors for me. His office was not far from my apartment and my work, which made it convenient for me to get regular check-ups. I took my medications – Lomotil and Salazapyrin – regularly. As I knew all too well, many Crohn's sufferers are troubled by the urgency of having to go to the bathroom, by cramps, and by diarrhea; Lomotil, an anti-diarrhea drug, helps to prevent such uncomfortableness and slows down the urgency to use the bathroom. But Lomotil is also a narcotic and its side effects include nausea, vomiting, drowsiness, and dizziness, and it can be addictive. Salazapyrin, which treats mild to moderate attacks of Crohn's disease or colitis and reduces the chances of flare-ups, was working well for me. Like most drugs, Salazapyrin also has side effects – nausea, reduced appetite, headaches, and allergic reactions such as rashes or swelling of the hands.

As I matured in my new job, I continued to experience new consequences of my Crohn's disease. I now felt like I was in Crohn's school – something new was thrown at me almost every day to learn. Although my health was fairly stable, in the middle of September I started to get headaches. I initially passed it off as tension headaches, hoping they would eventually go away. I put up with them for a while. However, they got worse and I could not concentrate at work. I went to see my doctor to get it checked out.

Dr. Conroy had left the province, so Dr. Mary Watson became my family doctor. It seemed that just as I got comfortable with one doctor, a new one came on the scene. As with most Crohn's sufferers, the number of doctors I was dealing with was unsettling. I had already told enough doctors my life story, I thought. However, I felt comfortable talking to Dr. Watson about my headaches. She suggested that the headaches were probably caused by Lomotil since this is one side effect of the drug. She suggested that I could go off Lomotil for a while and try another medication to address the diarrhea. But I had used other drugs, such as Imodium, before, and they were not as effective as Lomotil. Lomotil worked well for me, so I wanted to keep taking it if I could. Dr. Watson decided that reducing the amount of Lomotil I was taking might stop the headaches.

When I gave the pharmacist my prescription, he casually asked, "Why would a young girl like you be taking Lomotil?" I told him that

I had Crohn's disease. He nodded and replied, "Well, that's a good reason to be taking it." He told me that he had a friend who suffered from Crohn's disease and already had had about thirty bowel-related surgeries. I looked at the pharmacist in shock and wondered why he would want to tell me that. Maybe he just wanted to make conversation; I shrugged off his comments and thanked him for the pills.

A month passed and the terrible headaches persisted. I could not even bear the noise and voices at work. The least noise would worsen my headache. I managed to get through the pain until my next appointment with Dr. Higgins. I told him about my headaches; he suggested that Salazapyrin, not Lomotil, could be causing the headaches. Except for this, I was doing fairly well at this stage, so Dr. Higgins told me to stop taking Salazapyrin and to return to my normal dose of Lomotil. I was excited. The least amount of medication that I had to take sounded great to me. No more Salazapyrin.

I was happy that I was healthy enough to come off Salazapyrin; it was a good sign that I was slowly, but surely, becoming healthier. According to Dr. Higgins, why continue to take medication that could likely give me headaches if the Crohn's disease is already under control? This made complete sense to me. I walked out of his office that afternoon in good spirits. For the first time in a long time I was free of the main medication that I was taking specifically to keep my Crohn's disease at bay.

While this was a good sign, I wasn't totally free. A few weeks after my appointment with Dr. Higgins, I started to experience back pain. This was odd, as I had not experienced back pain before. I tried to remember if I had lifted anything that might have pulled a muscle. Maybe it was a pinched nerve that would go away in a day or two. Wishful thinking didn't work. The pain persisted and I felt miserable.

Sitting in the KIXX vehicle for three hours doing each morning show didn't help the situation, and I endured the pain for about a month. I was getting upset because I desperately wanted to be free of pain. It was frustrating: whenever I got over one hurdle, another popped up. All of these problems were the result of Crohn's disease. All I could think was, "I have had enough."

Being a Burden?

For a few weeks, I moped around at work, feeling tormented about my back pain. My co-workers asked what was wrong, as they obviously noticed that I was not acting like my usual self. I did not want to complain. I did not want to dampen their spirits; I didn't care about my own as I was good at handling that. But it would hurt to know that I was weakening the spirits of others. This often happens with Crohn's sufferers and people with any kind of chronic illness – you just don't want to bring anyone down with your complaining or the possible negative energy that might hover over you on the tough days. Most people who have a chronic illness try not to bring up their physical or emotional pain at work, and the last thing they want to do is complain.

But, as much as I hated to admit to my co-workers that I wasn't feeling well, I eventually had to tell them the truth. I knew they were sincerely concerned about me. I told them about my bad back, but I attempted to make light of the situation. Many times I suffered in silence and would never let on to anyone how much misery I was in as a result of my Crohn's. I did not want my co-workers to view me as a burden to the company. I sometimes felt isolated. My stomach ached every time I thought about what others might think of me. I wanted the ups and downs of this disease to end.

Around the end of November I told Dr. Higgins about my back pain. At first he thought it might be a slipped disc, but I knew I hadn't done anything to hurt my back or to pull a muscle. He suggested it might be inflammation, possibly in my spine. We talked about how Crohn's sufferers often get inflamed joints and experience arthritis-like conditions; it was similar to the conversation I had with Dr. Hewitt about my wrist and ankle joints a few months earlier. I prayed that I would never again have to experience such severe pain in my wrists and ankles. Inflamed joints are very painful, and I hoped that this bout would be short-lived. I saw this as another small hiccup in my recovery process, but I was determined not going to let an aching back keep me down. I was slowly gaining control of my Crohn's disease, so I wanted to drive over the bumps in front of me and keep on going.

Dr. Higgins said that if the symptoms worsened I should have tests done to determine the exact cause of the pain. The thought of having more tests was equivalent to asking me if I wanted needles stuck in my eyes. No more tests, I told him. He laughed.

CHAPTER SEVENTEEN

A Good Actor

*N*ovember was over, and another season of Christmas parties and receptions approached. It is a time when everybody seems happy, and people reflect on the importance of family and friends – something which I took seriously because of my family's vital role in helping me live with Crohn's.

My back still troubled me, but generally I was in good health. This was my first Christmas working in St. John's, and attending Christmas functions was a good chance for me to meet new people and to socialize with those I talked to almost every day on the phone but had never met in person, such as police officers, firefighters, politicians, and those who worked in the court system. It was a chance to do some networking.

While I was excited about mingling with new circles of people, Christmas socials meant food and alcohol. I was still cautious about the foods I ate, and alcohol sometimes gave me a bad stomach and caused diarrhea. To be safe, I always checked out bathroom locations in new surroundings. While everyone else indulged in food and sparkling drinks, I kept in mind the consequences I might face if I ate certain foods.

The best I could do, to be safe, was to nibble on a cracker, have a small piece of cheese, or maybe I'd be brave and eat a little salami or pepperoni and hope that I would not have to go to the bathroom. Sometimes I did eat more than I should, and, inevitably, pain followed. I became a genius at pretending that I had a friend across the room I wanted to greet, when, in fact, it was an escape to the bathroom. I prayed that nobody was behind me and that the bathroom was free. When I came out of the bathroom I held my head high – another successful simulation.

People often asked, "Why aren't you eating any of the food?" I was reluctant to tell them I couldn't eat because it made me have to use the bathroom. It was not easy to explain, and who wants to talk about a bowel disease at a social event? It seemed as though you could talk about cancer or diabetes and nobody had a problem discussing these illnesses, but bowel disease was off limits. This attitude often angered me.

Granted, I did not need alcohol to have a good time, but I would have enjoyed a social drink more without worrying about the consequences. It was frustrating not being able to enjoy food and alcohol like everyone else. There was, however, always Plan B – eat when I got home. When I arrived home after a function I usually ate too much. But I was in my own home, and I could use the bathroom as often as I needed to, without any embarrassment. If I had a pain in my stomach I could lie or sit down. My home became my refuge, a place where I did not have to worry about my condition.

Worsening Back Pain

I had a few days off at Christmas and I was excited about going back to Hare Bay and spending time with my family. I planned to leave St. John's on December 22 and return on Boxing Day. The night before I went home I awakened with a particularly sharp pain in my back. Dr. Higgins had told me to let him know if the pain increased. If I was going to experience back pain from time to time like this, when pain came without warning, then I wanted him to know about it. It hurt to lie in bed. It hurt to sit up. Even though I tried to stay away from the doctor's office as much as possible, I needed to call Dr. Higgins about my back.

I managed to get back to sleep. Before I knew it, my alarm went off – it was 4:30 a.m. I felt awful because of sleep deprivation and I could hardly move. My back was stiff and I knew I was in for a rough time driving around in the KIXX vehicle that morning. But it was my job and I had to persevere.

I arrived at work around 5:30 a.m. and did the morning traffic reports like any other day. It was three hours of misery. When I finished the morning show, I went back to the station and called Dr. Higgins. When I finally reached him, I told him that the back pain was not lessening and that I had hardly slept the previous night. I was going to Hare Bay that afternoon for Christmas, so I really wanted to get my back checked out before I left St. John's. Dr. Higgins was doing his rounds and could not see me himself, but he encouraged me to go to the emergency department and have a doctor examine me.

I told Brendan McCarthy that Dr. Higgins suggested I go to the hospital to get my back examined. Like always, Brendan was supportive, and he told me to take care of myself. Having an understanding boss made it less stressful and easier for me to deal with the daily challenges I faced living with Crohn's disease. I thanked Brendan for his concern, but my thanks had started to sound like apologies. For what? Because I was sick? The guilt would not give me a rest. I left work and went on the all-too-familiar drive to the Grace General Hospital. I arrived shortly after noon and headed to the emergency department. The lobby was full of people anxiously waiting to see a doctor. They looked restless and fidgety, and I knew I would have a long wait. I hated waiting, and it was even more difficult in a room full of sick people who looked glum. I managed to find a chair by the elevator. I sat down, stared at the ceiling, and thought that there had to be a better life waiting for me somewhere. Everyone in the room had a health problem, and I'm sure many of them were much worse off than me. But that didn't alleviate the pain and frustration I was going through. I was tempted to walk out of the emergency department and simply endure my distress.

A Heart-Warming Experience

But then, as I waited for my name to be called, I happened to glance at an old man sitting not far from me. I felt as though he had been staring at me. He had a warm, yet hesitant smile that created many lines across his forehead. He started to cough; I could tell he was in pain. I asked him if he needed some water, or if there was anything I could do for him. "No," he replied. I smiled, and started to look at a magazine. Then he said, "You can do one thing for me. You can promise that when you reach my age you'll always show off that smile because it makes others want to smile, too." I was taken aback by his comment. It touched my heart. "I promise," I replied. My heart ached for him being in the hospital all alone.

I continued to browse through magazines and became more and more impatient. All I could think was that these visits to hospitals to see a doctor are never over fast enough. For just once why couldn't I simply walk in a room, see a doctor, and walk out? It seemed as though I was always waiting. Life is too short to be stuck in waiting rooms, and, like most Crohn's sufferers, I was becoming a permanent fixture in doctors' offices and emergency departments. I felt sorry for myself. But as I ranted in my mind about the unfairness of the situation, I heard the old man's name called. This brought me back to reality. "Good luck," I said enthusiastically, as the nurse helped him walk across the room. Before he turned to go down the hall, he stopped and looked back at me. He smiled and walked away. A surreal feeling washed over me that afternoon – I wondered what would happen to him and if he would have any family with him for Christmas. I was glad I made him smile, as he seemed lonely and in need of a friendly face. I would never be alone, I thought. I had a family who loved me and many friends around me. No matter how sick I was, I would always have them to help me through. I felt differently about being in the emergency department that day. I believe that everything happens for a reason – on that day I brought a smile and a little joy into a lonely old man's life, and his presence was a physical reminder of how lucky I was to be surrounded by a caring family.

Sick of Hospitals

An hour passed. The waiting room was still crowded. Sitting on a hard and uncomfortable chair for a long time did not help my back. I got out of the chair to relieve some pressure. The nurse said I wouldn't have to wait too much longer. So much for dropping by the hospital and seeing a doctor right away! Maybe one day the hospital visits will get easier and move faster – that alone would make life easier for a Crohn's sufferer. I was in excruciating pain and I knew I wouldn't be able to do much when I arrived in Hare Bay, except rest.

Finally, it was my turn. By this time I also had a headache. The nurse led me to a room with two beds, one of which was occupied. I was given a Johnny gown to put on. I hated those thin, drafty gowns with the open backs. I felt unattractive and awkward wearing them, especially with so many people around. It wouldn't be so bad if I had a little privacy, but it was as if we were all lined up in jail attire waiting for our punishment. The gowns were too revealing, and I always felt vulnerable and humiliated when I had one on. But I had no choice – another matter beyond my control. Having to wear a Johnny gown once or twice in a lifetime for a medical procedure wouldn't be too much to complain about; but, like other Crohn's patients, always waiting in hospitals in a Johnny gown soon became an unpleasant, dreadful affair.

I had to provide a urine sample and then wait for somebody to see me. It wasn't long before the doctor on call was in the room. I described my back pain, and how at times the pain was unbearable. He examined me and asked some routine questions. I explained that I had Crohn's disease and that Dr. Higgins suggested I get my back checked out.

The doctor told me I had inflamed hip joints. He said this occurs in many Crohn's sufferers, and could become serious if not properly treated. If the problem is ignored, the inflammation might worsen and spread to other parts of the body. The drug used to treat this inflammation, Voltaren, could cause stomach problems, however. I was told to take two pills, three times a day, with my meals. He reminded me that if my stomach hurt at all, that I should advise my family doctor, and stop taking the drug. I prayed that this drug would help my back pain and not cause any dreadful stomach problems.

Before leaving for Hare Bay, I had my prescription filled. As I paid for the pills, the pharmacist looked at me and asked, "Aren't you a little young to be taking these pills?" I had heard this question before from another pharmacist when I had a Lomotil prescription filled. I told this pharmacist that I had joint pain as a consequence of Crohn's disease. He said he was used to filling such prescriptions for elderly people with arthritis. I didn't care who else took the drug; I simply wanted my back pain to end. I took two pills right away because I knew that sitting in one spot for almost four hours on the long ride home was going to be uncomfortable. I was already bent over because it hurt to straighten up. What a relief it was to finally see the Hare Bay sign. It would be good to have Mom take care of me.

CHAPTER EIGHTEEN

At Ease With Family and Friends

When I walked through the door, I could smell Mom's cooking. She had one of my favourite meals, homemade soup, waiting for me. Mom looked at me in amazement as I was so bent over. She lectured me about taking all of my medication and getting rest while I was home. She insisted that I obey doctor's orders. I thought, what would we do without mothers? The previous Christmas I had intense pain in my ankle and wrist joints and I spent most of my time in bed. I had hoped that every Christmas wasn't going to be like that.

I was so tired after supper that I was not up for visiting, so I called my friends and Nan Collins to let them know I was home and that I would visit them in the morning. I visited Dad that night, but it wasn't long before I went back to Mom's trailer to rest.

The medication relieved the back pain. After a few days, the Voltaren appeared to be working well and it did not cause any stomach problems. I was amazed at how fast the drug worked. I now felt more comfortable sitting and standing, and being free from the back pain was like someone had lifted a weight off my shoulders.

When I went home to Hare Bay everyone was cognizant of my illness. My discussions with people centred around how I was feeling, what foods I was eating, what medication I was on, and how I was coping at work.

On Christmas morning, Mom, my sister Dana, and I opened our gifts. Mom already had the turkey cooking for Christmas dinner, and the smell of turkey gave me a comforting feeling. While turkey was one of the foods that occasionally upset my stomach, I did not care that day; I was having turkey like everyone else.

I often joked that I never would have to worry again about getting fat because most foods I ate caused me to use the bathroom. I used to tell people that having Crohn's disease was a great diet. Even though

Mom knew I was joking, she still didn't like that comment. However, I had to deal with this frustrating illness my way, and joking about it was my way of accepting it. And I felt that when my family and friends joked with me it was their signal that it did not bother them that I had a bowel disease, so it shouldn't bother me either. I also realized that joking about my illness was a good way to educate people about it. At home, it became common for Mom or Dana to say, "Here she goes again," referring to the numerous times I'd get up from the table to use the washroom. We all laughed. We were free to have fun in our own home, without offending anyone. Everything seemed easier, more carefree, in Hare Bay.

The story was a little different when I ate at someone else's house. During Christmas, visiting neighbours and friends was a tradition in Hare Bay, and you weren't allowed to leave a house until you ate or had something to drink. I wasn't so quick to laugh if I felt the urge to use the bathroom then. I usually stuck with my eat-as-little-as-possible strategy – no food, no bathroom. Inevitably, however, someone would notice that I wasn't eating much. Then I'd have to pull excuses out of my hat – I wasn't hungry, or I ate before I arrived.

Before leaving Hare Bay for St. John's, I visited Lorelei's grave, a ritual whenever I returned home. I brought flowers. Each visit gave me a sense of peace, and the feeling that everything would be fine. As I knelt by her grave, my intended short update on my health and work turned into a dragged-out spiel. But I felt that she was listening.

By the time I went back to St. John's my back pain was gone, and I looked healthier, thanks to Mom's cooking and the new drug regime. I drove back with my friend Sheila and her fiancé; they were happy and in love. I envied them, especially at Christmas when, like many people, I am particularly sentimental. I was lucky to have such a loving family around me, but I lacked companionship. I looked forward to the day when I'd have a special man in my life – somebody by my side at all times, someone to confide in, to laugh with, to share my pain with, and to fight with over the bathroom!

CHAPTER NINETEEN

Unpredictable Flare-ups

I
t was the beginning of another year –1990. I prayed that this year
would bring me sustained good health. Work was going well and
I had many friends. However, my health was my sole focus. I wanted
the good days to continue; unfortunately, however, it seemed that
whenever things started to look up, something always happened to
crush my spirits.

One night in January, I awoke with severe abdominal pain. It was
so bad I did not know what to do. Should I call a friend? Should I go
to the hospital? I was alone and in excruciating pain. I was afraid to
go the hospital for fear of having to be admitted, so I got out of bed
and walked between the kitchen, the living room, and the bathroom.
The abdominal pressure was frightening. I bent over, holding my
stomach to ease the pain. I eventually crawled back into bed, crying.
I pressed a pillow against my stomach and finally fell asleep.

I dreaded such nights. I had had many of these episodes before I
was diagnosed with Crohn's disease. They always came out of the
blue – I never knew when the pain would hit. I would be quickly
whipped to a level of pain that seemed beyond endurance. Then, it
stopped as unexpectedly as it had begun. Even though my health,
overall, was good, thanks to surgery and medications, there were still
times when I experienced excruciating pain when I least expected it,
usually at night. I did not know why and, often times, doctors could
not explain it either. This time, however, it crossed my mind that the
bowel inflammation might have worsened because I was no longer
taking Salazapyrin, which had previously helped to get the Crohn's
under control, but it was also causing my headaches.

When my alarm went off a short time later, I hadn't gotten much
sleep. I was blurry-eyed. The pain lingered and I knew I was in no
condition to go to work, so I phoned my boss and told him I was sick.
I dreaded making the call. I felt guilty. Even though my illness was

legitimate, I always worried that someone might criticize me for being off work. I often had flashbacks to Gander and feeling like nobody believed I was sick. It was only natural that I sometimes felt uneasy, given what I had gone through there before I was diagnosed.

I knew I had a good support team at the KIXX radio station, but deep down I felt that some people still could not grasp the real pain and discomfort caused by Crohn's disease. I could not blame them for that. If, like them, I didn't have sleepless nights, chronic abdominal pain, aching joints, and constant trips to the bathroom, then I'd find it hard to understand. To truly appreciate what this horrible disease does to a person's everyday life, you have to experience it first-hand. While, for the most part, I had understanding co-workers, my work life was not perfect because of my occasional absenteeism, and, like most workplaces, there are always a few people who just don't under-stand, or don't care to understand. That's life. There will always be nay-sayers in the world, and nothing that we do or say will change their thinking. I could not deny that it hurt sometimes to think that someone might be talking about me and my illness in an ungracious manner, but I tried hard not to worry about it.

Being Thankful

While that feeling of uncertainty in terms of how people per-ceived me at work was often present in my mind, I decided to turn my energy towards positive things, such as how thankful I was for the help that I did receive from my on-air colleagues and other staff and management. I was especially grateful for their support of my volun-teer work with the St. John's chapter of the CFIC. The radio station helped us promote many fundraisers through free advertising on both Q-93 and KIXX FM stations and the company participated in events to raise money for IBD research. One memorable event was initiated by my KIXX FM morning show co-host Brian O'Connell. He did a live radio segment at a pizza restaurant in St. John's whereby he would go on air and encourage the public to buy a pizza in aid of Crohn's and colitis research – one dollar from every medium and large pizza sold was donated to the CFIC St. John's chapter. This sup-port from my workplace meant a great deal to me. It was as if my illness was being legitimized though such actions.

It is easier to forget about challenges when the people around you – co-workers, family, and friends – acknowledge that your illness is real. Any support that I received boosted my spirits and gave me hope that employers' support and understanding of challenges faced by employees with Crohn's would continue to increase as more people learned about IBD.

While I had a supportive work environment, my mind occasionally strayed to nasty thoughts of losing my job because of my illness. Even though I was determined not to let my illness ruin my career, I kept reminding myself that my health needed to be my number one priority. No job was worth sacrificing my health. Besides, if I didn't have good health, how would I be able to work?

After calling my boss that morning my guilt lingered as I waited for 9:00 a.m. to call Dr. Higgins. But it turned out that Dr. Higgins was on a leave of absence. Dr. Higgins had always been there for me when I was sick. I felt lost, and it hit me then how much I had relied on him to help me deal with my illness. Who would I rely on now?, I wondered.

I then phoned my family doctor in a panic because I was so sick and could not reach Dr. Higgins. Dr. Watson would see me that afternoon. While I had been sick like this many times before, each time still felt like the first time. I curled up on my bed and tried to rest while I waited for the time to go to the doctor's office. My friend Rodney, from the station, kept me company. Like many times before, his jokes distracted my pain.

I explained my episode of the previous night to Dr. Watson and told her that I needed something for pain. Dr. Watson suggested that I go back on Salazapyrin to reduce the inflammation in my bowel, and if the pain did not ease after a few days of taking the drug, I should see a bowel specialist. Several days passed and although I was feeling better and was back to work, I was still not back to my normal self. Despite my hesitation about seeing yet another doctor, the unbearable pain forced my surrender, and Dr. Watson referred me to another bowel specialist. My greatest fear was that the specialist, whom I would visit in the emergency department of the Grace General

Hospital, would tell me that I had to go back on steroids or be admitted to hospital for more tests.

All I could think was that as soon as I had recovered from the back pain, the abdominal pain returned. It became more tormenting, and, on top of that, I had to face another dreadful wait in an emergency department – the sterile surroundings and the hospital smell became all too familiar.

I put on my happy face as I braced for an encounter with yet another doctor. This specialist was a cheerful man who did not waste any time; he immediately asked me questions about my medical background, just as I had anticipated. I told him my life story in about ten minutes. (Every doctor in Newfoundland and Labrador must know my medical background by now, I thought.) The specialist examined me and ordered blood and urine tests; both, however, were normal. He believed I was experiencing another flare-up of Crohn's disease, and felt that Salazapyrin would be the best treatment for now, but he was adamant that if I became sick again I should immediately go to the hospital. I was exhausted after spending most of the day in the emergency department. I was sick and tired of being sick and tired. The only thing that doctors seemed to be able to do for me was to prescribe medication and order more tests.

On my way home I wished that my healthy days would last longer. I wanted to live as normal a life as possible. I wanted to be able to get through each day with the least amount of discomfort. I just wanted to work at building my career and spend time with my friends, like a normal person. Was this too much to ask?

CHAPTER TWENTY

Good Days and Bad Days

I continued to adapt to life with Crohn's disease in 1990 – taking my medications and obeying doctors' orders as best as I could. I got through spring without any major problems. It's amazing how sometimes I would feel so great that I would hardly notice that there was anything wrong with me. I looked and acted totally healthy.

Having Crohn's did not mean pain every day, but when I did feel sick, the pain was unbearable, and then I easily forgot the good days. I guess I should have been grateful for the good days, but I wanted to be cured.

I continued to work with the St. John's chapter of the CFIC. It has always been my hope that through the work of this foundation and the efforts of thousands of volunteers that a cure will be found for Crohn's disease. In the meantime, I knew we had to continue to enhance public awareness of IBD through whatever means possible. My role as the publicity chairperson of the St. John's chapter was an important one, and I was devoted to creating a greater awareness of IBD.

We utilized the media, including the provincial CBC TV program, "Coffee Break." The host of this program, Shirley Newhook, agreed to do a show on IBD. Ina Sheaves, who played a critical role in starting the St. John's chapter of the CFIC, as well as a gastroenterologist who was the chapter's medical advisor, and I would appear on the show. Ms. Newhook seemed genuinely interested in the work of the CFIC and its volunteers, and the show was another opportunity to inform the public of a support group for sufferers of Crohn's disease or colitis and to explain IBD and its treatment.

I survived the summer of 1990 without any major health problems. Other than going to the bathroom constantly, seeing my doctor on a regular basis, getting blood work done occasionally, and experiencing periodic bloating in my stomach, I was doing great. This was my life now, so I was determined to make the best of it. As long as I didn't have to go back on steroids or have more surgery, then I was relatively content.

The next time I got really sick again was mid-November. At 4:30 a.m. one morning, as I was getting ready for work, I suddenly felt weak. I stopped, sat on my bed, and put my hands on my head to prevent myself from fainting or throwing up. It was amazing how weak I was. I was still taking Lomotil to keep my diarrhea under control, especially when I knew I would be out in public. Despite taking Lomotil when I felt I needed it, I still had problems with diarrhea. I believed that the sporadic bouts of diarrhea (sometimes I went to the bathroom ten and twelve times a day) was taking a toll on me. Having constant diarrhea would probably make any person weak, given that it would likely result in the loss of essential vitamins and nutrients.

Feeling sick before I went to work in the mornings had a tremendous emotional effect on me, and work was the first thing I thought of every time I became sick. I always felt guilty when sickness prevented me from working. There were times when I even thought, was it all in my head?

With this current painful bout of Crohn's, I needed to see my family doctor as soon as possible. A few weeks later I saw a specialist; I told him about my weak spells, like the one of a few weeks earlier, the constant diarrhea, and various other symptoms. We talked about my work situation – new management, major changes, anticipated lay-offs.

Worrying about work might have played a minor role in the recent bout of sickness and increased trips to the bathroom. Even normal healthy people often go to the bathroom more frequently when they are nervous or worried. For Crohn's sufferers, this is even more pronounced. The doctor ordered more tests, including X-rays and blood work. I had to request time off work to get the tests done the next day. I dreaded to ask for more time off. My next appointment would be a week later to discuss the results of my tests.

The night before the tests I had to drink an entire bottle of Citro-mag, a laxative that would clean out the bowel before I could have the X-ray. Citro-mag tasted awful. It was not the first time I had drunk it, but, like everything else associated with Crohn's, it does not get easier. The colder the drink, the easier it was to swallow; nausea and cramping typically followed ingestion.

I had yet another long wait at the hospital the next morning. I was getting impatient, as I sat in a chair with my blue Johnny gown on – again – and people walking up and down the halls looking at me. What a sight I was – wearing a blue hospital gown and my socks and boots.

What a life for a young woman, I thought. Like always, most people in the room were older than me, the average age was sixty. I felt like an old woman full of aches and pains.

I was finally called in. I recognized the X-ray technicians from previous visits and joked with them, saying how we'd soon be on a first-name basis.

The next few days before going back to see my specialist, Dr. Higgins, were nerve-racking because I was afraid of what would show up on the X-rays. This fear popped up each time I waited for test results. When I walked into Dr. Higgins's office, I wanted the verdict right away, and I got it. The X-rays showed some swelling in my bowel near the area of the bowel re-section. Although the swelling didn't appear to be serious, we talked about my going back on steroids to prevent it from getting worse. This was not something that I was receptive to, given my previous experience with steroids. Dr. Higgins wanted to run another test before he made a final decision. He gave me a prescription for Prednisone anyway, but told me not to fill it until he had the results from a second test. I hesitantly put the prescription in my handbag. Dr. Higgins knew I detested steroids.

Nightmares of my Prednisone use in the past came rushing back. I felt distressed just thinking about the negative experiences I had already had with the drug: bloating, swelling, sweating, etc. Why would God put me through that again?

I was also not pleased about more X-rays. This time, it was an Upper GI Series. Dr. Higgins also told me I had to resume monthly B_{12} injections. I had been taking B_{12} shots off and on since my diagnosis. The results of my latest blood work showed a low B_{12} count, a factor which contributed to my weakness.

I was nervous at work for the next few days while I waited for the results of the Upper GI Series. I prayed for good results. Most of my anxiety was over having a setback. I had been doing fairly well for almost a year and then, out of the blue, I was faced with the possibility of going back on steroids.

I waited for Dr. Higgins to call, but knew that if I did not hear from him it was likely that nothing alarming had showed up in the X-rays. I was relieved to have gotten through Christmas without experiencing any further health problems.

With another new year, 1991, came the talk of more resolutions. I had no intention of making any. Like most people, I somehow managed not to keep them. But I made one wish every year: to have good health. I prayed that 1991 would be my healthiest year ever.

My next scheduled appointment with Dr. Higgins was January 9. This Christmas holiday was a far cry from the previous Christmas and New Year's when I had been suffering from a bad back and the one before that when I had aching wrists and ankles. Dr. Higgins did not contact me over the holidays, so I assumed my check-up had been fine.

In the new year I received good news. At my next appointment, Dr. Higgins informed me that the second X-ray showed only a minor bowel irritation. Nothing, according to him, that would warrant putting me back on Prednisone. I was ecstatic, and hoped that the minor irritation would not worsen. Hearing that I did not have to go back on steroids gave me greater hope that my progress would continue.

MICHELLE PHILLIPS
GOULDS
AGE: 15

I was diagnosed with Crohn's disease in May 2002 at the age of twelve. Before I was diagnosed, I felt horrible. I was going to the bathroom about seven or eight times a day. Every time I ate I would get vicious pains in my stomach, sometimes I fell over in pain. I was living like that for about two months before I was sent to see a specialist in March 2002. I was finally "officially" diagnosed with Crohn's disease in May 2002. The hardest part of being sick was missing school. I absolutely hated missing school and falling behind.

After I was diagnosed, I was put on steroids and other pills. We tried many methods – different pills, medicine – to keep my disease under control; the trials and errors seemed endless. I always remember how I just wanted the pain to stop. Finally in October 2004, we stumbled upon something that worked: NG (nasogastric) tube feedings. It wasn't easy going everywhere with a "stupid" tube hanging out of my nose – it was sometimes unbearable. I was torn between feeling better physically, and feeling much worse emotionally. What was also so hard was having to go without food.

After I realized I could not be taken off the feedings I got a G tube – a tube that went into my stomach from my abdomen. After a while of being on feedings at night and eating during the day I got worse and worse. Finally, during the summer of 2005 I was put on the dreaded steroid called Prednisone. This worked for a short while. I eventually started throwing up everything I ate; my stomach blew up and I resembled a pregnant woman. When Prednisone didn't work and the vomiting persisted, I was hospitalized. After further testing, it was discovered that I had a blockage. At that time surgery was the only alternative. I had one-half of my large bowel and a small portion of my small bowel removed in

September 2005. I am still on various medications and tube feedings. Since my surgery I have gained weight and grown a little. I am feeling really well and getting some normalcy back in my life. I am also doing really well in school. I miss very little school now, and I even joined the Cheerleading team! My wish for the future is that I will not have to have any more surgery and that things will get back to normal, whatever that "normal" will be.

CHAPTER TWENTY-ONE

Accepting My Illness

The weeks and months following my appointment with Dr. Higgins in January 1991 were good ones. I went around like someone who had never experienced pain. I continued to enjoy my work in radio and missed fewer days because of my Crohn's. I felt healthy and optimistic about my future. I was especially glad for finding the strength to hold my head high during the emotional pain of learning to live with IBD, which can, at times, be more burdensome than the physical pain. Crohn's disease can be embarrassing for some people, and, given the nature of the illness, they often hide it from others; they bottle up their frustrations and often deal with it alone, which can be mentally draining and upsetting. While I felt upset and frustrated many times having to cope with Crohn's, I made a decision not to let pride get in my way of being open about my illness, and never to let guilt drag me down.

I continued to hear more stories about other people suffering from IBD. I was surprised by the number of people who were either suffering from this disease or knew someone who was. While I did not think it was possible, I learned that many sufferers experienced worse pain than I had, and some people's experiences with Crohn's were far more devastating and alarming than mine.

As I continued to get stronger and get my illness under control, I became resigned to the fact that I could not change how things were, and pledged to myself to fight this disease. I was getting back to a more normal life as each year passed, and I believed my focus now was to try and turn my experience into something positive. I focused on doing more to raise an awareness of IBD. I wanted to help others who needed someone to talk to or needed to be reminded that they were not alone. I believed in the value of doing small things that make a big impact, such as talking about the disease and reaching out to other sufferers in whatever forum possible.

As time went on, my involvement with the CFIC's St. John's chapter became a greater priority. I continued as publicity chairperson for a few years, and I was passionate about my volunteer commitment.

Speaking Out About Crohn's

In November 1991, I received a phone call from Emily Dyckson, the lifestyles editor of *The Evening Telegram* newspaper, requesting an interview with me about living with Crohn's disease. Given that November was Crohn's and colitis public awareness month, she wanted to talk to me about my battle with IBD. I agreed because I saw this as an opportunity to educate people about this challenging disease, which can affect anyone at any age.

I was proud to speak publicly about my illness through such a forum and let others who suffered from Crohn's know that they are not alone in suffering from this disease. I was no longer ashamed to talk about my pain and bowel troubles. The specifics of Crohn's disease is not an attractive topic, but I was determined to help erase the stigma of IBD and influence people's views towards the illness.

Dyckson's feature article did help to change some people's attitudes. I received many phone calls from people who were either suffering from IBD or had a friend or family member who was. I also received phone calls from people who did not suffer from the disease, but who, after reading the article, felt compelled to contact me and wish me luck. One person told me I was a brave woman. I do not consider myself brave; I am just someone trying her best to live a normal life – as normal as a Crohn's sufferer could – while also trying to help others who suffer from the disease.

The response to the article was uplifting, and I was touched by the kind words. Most importantly, I was pleased that the article had generated much-needed discussions about IBD. I believed that the disease deserved public and media attention, like any other serious illness.

I hoped that in the days, months, and years ahead the discussion about IBD would continue. I also hoped that one day bowel disease would be part of our common conversation, like diabetes, cancer, or kidney disease. Above all, I wanted the silence that surrounded IBD to cease.

The beginning of Emily Dyckson's article has particular resonance: "Looking at Sonia Glover no one would guess that life has been a continuous battle of pain and suffering. She looks the picture of health." One thing I have noticed, as I am sure other Crohn's sufferers do, when people find out that I have Crohn's disease they are usually surprised. The typical response that I receive is "I'd never know there was anything wrong with you, especially with your bubbly personality. Sure, you look great." Why do people think that if you have an illness you have to look a certain way? Anyone can look good on the outside, but that doesn't mean they are healthy.

An Uplifting Reunion

As I tried to live as normal a life as possible, I often thought about Jane Ball, the nurse who had been so kind and cheerful when I was hospitalized for bowel surgery. I thought about her during my many visits to emergency departments. One day, about two years after my surgery, I was at a going-away party for a relative who was leaving the Grace General Hospital to work outside of the province. When I arrived at the party, a woman was walking down the stairs in the foyer. I knew we had met before, but I could not remember where. She also looked at me as if to say "I know you from somewhere" when I approached her. She said her name was Jane Ball and she was a nurse at the Grace General Hospital. When I told her my name, she remembered me. But she was amazed at how much I had changed. Jane reminded me that she had seen me at my worst when I was in the hospital. She could not believe how healthy I looked. That night I had a glow on my face – quite a contrast to my white and "sick" face. My hair was a different style, I had extra make-up on my face, and I was dressed up. I looked great and felt great.

Jane and I soon realized that we lived only a few minutes from each other in downtown St. John's. We reminisced about my time in the hospital – the pain and the laughter. We made plans to get together for coffee and, after that, we became good friends. Jane and her family eventually moved to Nova Scotia. I believe that something good always comes out of something bad – Jane's friendship is proof of this. If I had not had bowel surgery at the Grace General Hospital in January 1988, I probably would never have been blessed with her friendship. Nineteen years later, Jane and I still keep in touch.

CHAPTER TWENTY -TWO

Staying Positive Works

I have learned that people's experiences with Crohn's disease vary. Some individuals' pain and torment are worse than others. For many Crohn's sufferers drug therapy is sufficient. For others, one surgery is effective to keep the disease under control. Others require several surgeries and the battle is continuously uphill. While there are many different conditions and situations associated with Crohn's, there is one common denominator – pain.

Besides medical treatments, I believe the gradual and steady improvement in my health after 1991 was aided by my positive attitude. I described it as my anchor, with my supportive family and friends playing critical roles. They were there to give me an extra nudge on my toughest days.

My continued work with the St. John's chapter (renamed Eastern Avalon Chapter) of the CFIC (renamed Crohn's and Colitis Foundation of Canada [CCFC]), remained an integral part of my life; it helped me accept my illness and be proud of who I am. I remain a volunteer with the CCFC Eastern Avalon Chapter today, and I am honored to be part of such a worthy cause. My almost twenty years as a CCFC volunteer has enriched my life and has enabled me to keep things in perspective.

Given all of the frustration and pain I went through as a young woman trying to get her career off the ground, and after difficult months of turmoil early on in my career, my illness has never held me back. I have managed to cope well. Each year was better than the previous one and I was fortunate not to have any serious flare-ups. Despite a few scares, I did not have to go back on Prednisone after my bowel surgery. I pray that I never will.

For a while, the many doctors' visits and tests continued. Besides the usual Upper GI Series and Barium Enema, I also had to undergo a colonoscopy, a test dreaded by just about every Crohn's sufferer that

I have met. I was heavily sedated for this procedure, where a long flexible tube was inserted through my rectum into my intestine to examine my colon. My sister Dana and friends Melinda and Randy came to the hospital with me. I was extremely nervous and it was the most nerve-racking procedure I've ever had. The hardest part of it for me, and for most patients, was the preparation – the bowel has to be completely cleaned out before the test can be performed, to ensure the doctor gets the best view of the colon. A rectal examination is also done prior to the colonoscopy. The thought of a rectal exam always made me cringe. After the test, Melinda teased me about the gibberish I was speaking when they were waiting for me to wake up. She joked that I had learned a new language.

I knew that my health was getting better, and while the colonoscopy was not particularly appealing, I didn't mind the various medical procedures in the short term; I simply got used to them. Having Crohn's disease means I likely will have to undergo a colonoscopy periodically for the rest of my life.

For me, having Crohn's simply became syonymous with everyday challenges and frustrations. I knew that I couldn't just click my fingers and make the disease disappear, so I plugged along and tried to make each day as productive as possible. I kept a positive outlook and woke up every morning hoping that each day would be better than the previous one.

Committed to My Career

As my health improved, my priority was to work hard at building my career, and to always be as professional as I could be. Besides radio, I worked in newsprint as a reporter and photographer, I freelanced for different publications, and in the mid-1990s I moved into the exciting world of public relations.

In all of my jobs after radio, including the *Mount Pearl Post* newspaper, Memorial University of Newfoundland, and the provincial government, I still had occasional bad days due to my illness, but I got past them, thanks to my determination and supportive colleagues. Indeed there were days when I felt like crying out of frustration, but many others when I felt like laughing my head off from being in such ridiculous situations, like the times I sat on the toilet in a bathroom at work keeping my feet off the floor when someone came in so they would not know it was me, or days when I heard someone complain about the smell of perfume in the bathroom or they thought someone had been smoking in the bathroom (which was prohibited), when, in fact, I had lit a match or sprayed the cheap perfume to mask the foul smell.

It didn't matter where I worked, Crohn's disease was ever-present. While the work environments changed, the pain and frustration remained the same. As time went on, I decided not to spend my valuable time worrying about my health. I realized that my health really wasn't all that terrible.

I am proud of my strong work ethic; I possess a great passion for work – some friends even call me a workaholic. I often wonder if my extreme passion for work resulted from being unable to work in 1987, the year I was diagnosed with Crohn's. I still find it upsetting that the illness took away my job for a short period of time. It was an overwhelming and sad time in my life. I had no control, which may be why I absorb myself in work all of the time. I am happy and fortunate to have done what I have always wanted to do, despite my health issues, and that is to work in the communications field, whether in journalism or public relations.

Crohn's and Stress

From time to time, theories about the cause of Crohn's disease arise, especially the relationship between stress and flare-ups of the disease. Personally, I do not believe there is a link. I was a Director of Communications for the provincial government for over seven years and worked with many cabinet ministers in various departments. Having this job meant long working hours, sometimes seven days a week, involving extensive multi-tasking, and a fast-paced and high-pressure environment. This is the nature of politics. While this made for stressful days, I did not experience a single flare-up while I was in this position. In fact, I did not lose a day because of Crohn's disease, other than for regular check-ups or specific medical tests. And I very rarely did that – I am ashamed to admit that I actually had a habit of missing doctors' appointments because I was too busy at work. I was often stubborn when it came to my health, which resulted in frequent lectures from my friends, family, and colleagues.

I've disagreed with people who suggest that anyone with Crohn's disease cannot or should not work in a highly stressful environment. Every Crohn's sufferer is different, and, depending on their symptoms and the status of their illness, people make choices – some choose to stay away from stressful environments for fear that it might impact them, others are not bothered by high pressure situations and learn how to manage the stress and their Crohn's. Indeed I am proof that even people involved in highly stressful environments can control the disease and perform duties effectively. While it is not so much the case today, if you mentioned Crohn's disease years ago, most people would automatically link it to stress. If someone is stressed, it doesn't matter what illness they have, the stress will likely exacerbate it – but stress shouldn't only be associated with Crohn's.

I will never forget a conversation I had in 1989 with Dr. Sean Conroy. One day, during a check-up, we were discussing my line of work, how I got into radio, and how busy I was. He noted how stress had been connected to IBD. Although the relationship between stress and IBD had not been proven conclusively at the time, and is still not today, Dr. Conroy suggested then that I might not be able to stay in radio forever due to the fast pace of the media business, the tight deadlines, and the associated stress. The conversation surprised me at the time, and, for several days after this discussion I was paranoid, thinking he was trying to prepare me for something horrible in connection with my job; maybe my illness would cause me to lose my job. I came to the conclusion, however, that Dr. Conroy had no hidden messages that day. He was simply trying to point out that some jobs have more stressors than others; this is an important factor for anyone to consider when deciding on a career path, especially if he or she suffers from a serious illness. But as far as I was concerned, it depends on how we manage job stress and life's challenges. This has been the case for me in all of my jobs. I was always determined not to let Crohn's disease impede my career; and I was certainly not going to let stress hold me back.

The Family Perspective:

FRANCES GLOVER
MOTHER OF SONIA B. GLOVER
HARE BAY

When I look back at Sonia as a young child, I remember a very sick little girl who turned into a sick young woman. It started as a tummy ache. She always had a pain in her stomach. Like most mothers, I thought that maybe my child wanted to stay out of school – that was my first reaction. My young daughter would always have severe pain in her stomach and sides. She was miserable and there was nothing I could do. I took her to the doctor many times, but the answer I always got was, "there is nothing wrong with your little girl," or the doctor would list all the maybes – maybe it was stomach flu, maybe it was bowel spasms, maybe it was a urinary tract infection, maybe it was all in her mind – that's what I had to deal with.

I remember the times when Sonia's teachers would call me and say, "Please come and get your daughter, and don't bring her back to school until you take her to a doctor." What was I to do? I was very stressed; I felt helpless watching my daughter suffer. Sonia constantly cried from abdominal cramps, and threw up almost everything she ate. One vivid memory is of seeing her head over the toilet bowl, always vomiting. I recall the nights she cried out from her bedroom and I would turn on the radio, which helped her fall asleep. We were eventually told she had a stomach ulcer, and she was given medication. But the pain did not stop.

Sonia dealt with her sickness in her own way. She graduated from high school and then went on to graduate from the journalism program at Bay St. George Community College in Stephenville. In Stephenville, it was the same thing all over again – she was sick all the time. I was so far away from her, I could not help. I wanted to be by her side and try to ease her pain. All I could think was I would rather that I was sick myself, not her. During college she ended up in Gander hospital, going through a rough time once more. She was so very sick. It broke my heart to see her in so much pain and agony. I watched her in pain and felt it myself.

Finally, Sonia was diagnosed with Crohn's disease. I remember accompanying her to St. John's – she had to be admitted to hospital for surgery. It was a worrisome time for me as a mother. And, it was frightening for her as a young woman, when she didn't know what to expect. I remember the specialist talking to us about the surgery and explaining there was always a possibility that Sonia would need a colostomy. This truly was a nightmare. Sonia underwent surgery and had a portion of her bowel removed. A colostomy was not necessary. It was great news. And, I know it was playing on Sonia's mind. I remember so clearly when she woke up after surgery, the first thing she did was put her hand down by her side to see if she had a colostomy or ileostomy.

I remember Sonia having to take some time off work due to her sickness. I was very worried when she was on sick leave. I knew how important a career was to her. I could see that it bothered her being off work. Again, it was out of my control. I felt helpless. Sonia had many ups and downs with her sickness, but it never affected her like I thought it would. She learned to accept her illness and cope with it. She also helped other people with the disease, which made me very proud as a mother. My daughter has made great progress, and I know her Crohn's will never hold her back. She is a fighter, but sometimes I think she works too hard – that's my opinion. There are also times when I know she doesn't take care of herself like she should, and that worries me a lot. And, I know that she still has some bad days, but she won't admit it.

Also, as a mother I have a constant worry because I know that Sonia will always have Crohn's disease. I cannot bear the thought of seeing her go through so much suffering again. Regardless of what the future holds, I'll be there for Sonia. I will be her pillar of strength. Through it all, I am extremely proud of my daughter, that she fought this battle head-on, and many times she did it all alone. Sonia once said, "Mom, you can either be on a wheel and keep spinning around and around and go nowhere, or you can get off that wheel and move forward." I'll never forget that comment. Sonia had the willpower to keep moving forward – she had the guts!

CHAPTER TWENTY-THREE

Finding Love

As a Crohn's sufferer, the idea of having a serious relationship
with someone who understood my illness was always a frightening thought. How difficult would it be to find someone who would not
be embarrassed by such a disease? What if, in the middle of a romantic, candlelight dinner, I had to suddenly rush to the bathroom because
of diarrhea? These questions haunted me for a while after I was diagnosed. I did not want to repulse a date or some guy that I might be
interested in. Many people cannot cope with a partner who is afflicted with a chronic illness, certainly not a bowel disease like Crohn's.
Rejection is always a possibility.

While most of my friends wondered if their parents would like
their boyfriends, I wondered if I would even find a boyfriend who
would not be disgusted by my bowel disease. Bowel disease sounded
so ugly and repugnant.

While I did not let Crohn's disease keep me from dating and experiencing short-term relationships, I still felt uneasy about having
Crohn's. I always worried about finding someone with whom to share
my life, someone who wouldn't be embarrassed or uncomfortable
about my illness over the long term. Not knowing what the future
could bring for my illness could have an impact on commitment and
be considered too much "baggage" to even start a relationship. If the
shoe were on the other foot, I think I, too, would have to think long
and hard before committing to a serious relationship with someone
who had a major health issue. Dealing with an illness such as Crohn's
can result in instant stress for someone starting a new relationship.
This was more so years ago, because of a lack understanding about
IBD; but even today many people know little about Crohn's disease
and it is still not talked about like other diseases.

I often found it difficult to imagine a guy who would want to
bring me to meet his parents and have to say, "Hi Mom and Dad, meet

the love of my life. Isn't she beautiful? Oh, and by the way, she has inflammatory bowel disease." Besides wondering if I would ever find a life-long soul mate, early on in my illness I always feared the thought of parents whispering to their son, "Of all the girls you could be with, why did you have to choose someone with an illness like Crohn's?" And if I was in a serious relationship, there was the recurring fear about the impact my Crohn's could have on me or my partner during intimacy. What if I lost control of my bowels? How would my partner or husband feel? How would I handle it? As I was still learning and trying to cope with Crohn's, all of these scenarios crossed my mind.

Just knowing that I had Crohn's disease sometimes made me feel unattractive and dirty. Did others see me that way? While many of my fears seemed far-fetched to some people, they existed for me. Many people with Crohn's experience the same fears, especially early on in their illness.

But paranoia completely disappeared in 1995 when I met Paul Sullivan. Paul and I soon discovered that we had much in common – we came from broken homes, we were passionate about our work, we loved to exercise, and we enjoyed a good joke. I thought we were a perfect match and were meant to be together forever.

I immediately told Paul that I had Crohn's disease, as I thought it was just as well to get it over with. I was relieved when it became clear that my illness was not an issue for Paul. In fact, he was intrigued and wanted to learn more about the illness and the struggle I had endured before we met. Paul has never seen me go through the kind of excruciating pain I experienced around the time I was diagnosed with Crohn's – I hope he never does.

As our relationship grew, Paul often spent nights at my apartment and those were the times when I wished Crohn's was out of my life. While Paul knew I had this disease, and he was sympathetic, I don't think he realized how it had affected my life. I always wore my typical happy face and kept upbeat, and on the outside it didn't look like there was anything wrong with my health.

Hiding My Illness

By the time I met Paul my disease was well under control. I didn't experience constant stomach pain, but I was still going to the bathroom quite frequently. Thinking that I might offend Paul by my frequent visits to the bathroom, I often resorted to my not-eating tactic. If I did not eat, there was a good chance I would not experience diarrhea.

I also tried to schedule my bowel movements for the times when Paul was not around, and, when he was at my apartment, I did what I could to keep from going to the bathroom. This is difficult to do if you have Crohn's, and I soon discovered it was not wise as it created extra pressure on my already abnormal bowel, causing more pain. Generally, physicians say that holding bowel movements could cause a weakening of the anal sphincter, which is the muscle at the end of the digestive track that keeps the stool inside.

Because I awoke many times in the middle of the night to use the bathroom when Paul stayed with me, I often tried to hold the diarrhea for fear of waking him. I wanted to avoid exposing him to the sometimes embarrassing smell and noise my bowels made when I used the bathroom. Many nights I crept into the bathroom, praying that Paul would not hear me. I would light several matches to get rid of the foul smell and I became adept at having a bowel movement in portions, letting just a little bit of stool out at a time to reduce the noise. I suffered pain in my belly as I did this, but at the time I was desperate not to expose Paul to that detail of the disease.

It was embarrassing for me, and I just did not want to deal with it early in our relationship. And I would go through great lengths to avoid it. Many times I cleaned the bathroom all over – sink, vanity, toilet, and tub – with a strong cleaner to freshen it up before I came out. Cleaning the bathroom from top to bottom would always do the trick to get rid of the unpleasant smell.

As time went on and our relationship grew stronger, I realized that I was more worried about Paul's response to my having Crohn's than he was. It was my issue, not Paul's. Paul was not disgusted by my Crohn's; he just wanted me to be healthy.

Paul and I were married in 1999. Brian O'Connell emceed the

reception and told many stories about when we worked together at KIXX FM. Even though I was often sick back then, Brian still remembered the fun moments; it was heart-warming to hear these anecdotes on my wedding day. Today Paul and I often crack jokes with each other about my Crohn's. Sometimes, it is actually very funny, such as when I am in the washroom and Paul yells out, "Is it safe to come in there now?" And then I open the bathroom door and we both burst into laughter. I continue to look for the humour in everything – it keeps life simple and fun. And, one thing that keeps us both happy is that we do not have to fight over the bathroom – there are three in our home! As Paul says, jokingly, "It's a good thing we do!"

Adapting comfortably to life with Crohn's disease is not possible without the support of family and friends, and it is important to have an understanding employer. I have been fortunate to have had such support over the years. I am blessed with a wonderful husband, a family who love me, and a large circle of caring friends. Without them I would not have been able to fight this illness and live my *almost normal* life today.

CHAPTER TWENTY-FOUR

Living Healthy and Happy with Crohn's

Today, almost twenty years after my diagnosis, my Crohn's is still active. However, I have had no major flare-ups in several years and hope I never do. I have fully accepted that I have Crohn's disease and am not ashamed of it. My feelings of isolation and frustration that were frequent years ago because of the impact that Crohn's was having on my everyday life have disappeared. While I wish I did not have the disease, I no longer let it upset me. I remind myself every day that my health issues are minor compared to the challenges that some people face.

Having active Crohn's means I continue to have days when the number of trips I make to the bathroom can't be counted on one hand, between a half-dozen and a dozen times on most days. I still have occasional discomfort in my stomach, but nothing so severe that I can't handle; most times it's a diet issue. I am also B_{12} deficient and continue to take B_{12} needles monthly; and I still experience aches and pains in my joints from time to time. I don't vomit anymore after I eat, for which I am extremely grateful.

I also have had sporadic bouts of memory loss over the years. There were times when I was so scared and frustrated with my poor memory that I thought that I might be getting dementia. I had some tests done, including a memory test, and everything appears fine. However, some research shows a link between B_{12} deficiency and neurological symptoms like poor memory, so maybe that could be a factor in my memory problems. My family doctor is aware of my concern and the issue will continue to be monitored. There are, of course, many people who simply don't have a good memory, and maybe I am one of them.

Despite all of these minor discomforts, I feel healthy and am extremely happy with my life. Considering all of the pain and suffering that I endured before I was diagnosed with Crohn's and the months following my diagnosis, trying to understand the dimensions of the illness, I feel blessed today. God has been good to me and I am fortunate to live a good life, even with Crohn's disease. I now eat almost anything I want. Certain foods, particularly those that are starchy and greasy, could pose problems, so I often avoid those. Sometimes I eat these foods anyway, despite the potential consequences. I drink a lot of fresh milk; it still does not bother my stomach (many IBD sufferers have a lactose intolerance). I still love bologna and, while I know processed food is not healthy, I eat it occasionally: I fry it and I pour ketchup on it; it tastes delicious and it does not give me a bad stomach!

I admit that I like to splurge every now and then, but, for the most part, I am a healthy eater and I exercise. I believe a balanced diet and regular exercise are important whether or not you suffer from an illness. Exercising almost every day and eating well have had a positive impact on my health – it makes me feel better, both physically and mentally.

While joint and stomach pains exist for me, they are limited compared to years ago, and I rarely talk about it – I just deal with it. Besides, who wants to listen to someone complain all the time? Complaining is certainly not going to make it better. I have learned to adapt and have fun in the process. For me, coping is all about the little things, like timing my meals. If I am going to a social function, I try to eat early enough so that if I need to make an urgent trip to the bathroom it will be taken care of before I leave home. Alternatively, I may eat something that I know will not negatively affect me, or I don't eat at all and wait until I return home. Being on an anti-diarrhea drug eliminates this concern for most Crohn's sufferers. I avoid taking medication whenever I can, so instead of taking Lomotil, I now eat lots of grapes – yes, not only are they a healthy fruit, they are the best anti-diarrhea treatment for me. From time to time, I also take an off-the-shelf anti-diarrhea medication, Imodium, mostly when I travel, especially if I am travelling to a less-developed country. I will continue to eat grapes if it means staying off medication to control diarrhea, and it doesn't negatively impact my health (I've discovered that eating too many grapes at once can cause constipation). I always ensure that my family doctor is aware of my home remedies.

Mouthwash and toothpaste still hurt my stomach from time to time and cause me to use the bathroom. Mouthwash gives me the greatest discomfort; I use it at least a half hour before I leave home in the mornings, or if I go out in the evenings, which leaves enough time for me to visit the bathroom if I need to.

Then, there are matches. I don't know what I would do without them. I still carry matches in my handbag and I even keep them in my bathrooms at home, along with numerous home fragrances, scented candles, and containers of baby wipes to freshen up after using the bathroom. Over the years, using matches for this purpose has created amusing and memorable times with my girlfriends. Making sure one of us had matches was a critical part of getting ready for a night out. We laughed hard some nights in a public bathroom while one of us was lighting the match as another kept watch. And there was always the little bottle of perfume that one of us had in our handbags that we could rely on if the matches failed. My friends were good sports like that, always making light of the situation, which made me feel better about having Crohn's. We actually had fun because of my illness; it all made for some special memories.

Crohn's sufferers discover their own effective coping mechanisms. And they learn early on that in addition to the physical impact of the disease, the mental and emotional effects are equally challenging.

Live for the Day

I don't know whether the days of my extreme pain and discomfort will return. The doctors don't know. Crohn's disease is like a ghost hiding around the corner. If and when it pops out, I will deal with it, with the help of my husband, family, and friends. While flareups of Crohn's disease are unpredictable, I remain optimistic that the worst of my illness is over. I fully recognize that Crohn's is a serious and chronic disease; however, I feel confident that I will continue to live a full and enjoyable life with it.

More advanced treatments and new medications are available for IBD sufferers today than when I was diagnosed. Salazapyrin, the drug that I was prescribed in the 1980s, has been replaced with more effective drugs – Asacol, Pentasa, Imuran, Methotrexate, and Remicade. With such a variety of drugs and more advanced treatments now available, many IBD sufferers are better able to cope with their illness and live more productive lives.

There was a time when I wondered if Crohn's was the cause of my sickness when I was growing up. And, if so, why did it take so long to diagnose? My mother often posed this question. If I had been diagnosed earlier, maybe I would not have had gone through so much pain and humiliation in college, or maybe the suffering and frustration in my first full-time job could have been reduced or avoided altogether.

Today, I do not dwell on the what-ifs. I still believe that God has a purpose for all of us, and I view life as a precious journey. I am determined to enjoy the journey each and every day. As a Crohn's sufferer, it's simple – I make the best of my good days and get through the tough days by thinking about the good days.

In light of the consequences that come with having Crohn's disease, I feel that I am a stronger person, and I will use that strength to help others, as well as to deal with any other of life's challenges. My experience has taught me to enjoy life, to see the good in all people, and be grateful for everything I have. After all, it could always be worse.

While coping with Crohn's has taught me many things about life and happiness, two important lessons stand out – I never take my health for granted, and it's not about what happens to me in life, it's what I choose to do about it.

In the end, laughter, a positive attitude, and perseverance will always pull you through, no matter what the illness or challenge in life. It has worked for me.

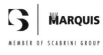

MEMBER OF SCABRINI GROUP

Québec, Canada
2007